Code to Care

Code to Care

A Leaders' Guide to Implementing Responsible AI in Healthcare

Rubin Pillay MD PhD

Copyright © 2024 by Rubin Pillay MD PhD.

Library of Congress Control Number:		2024900751
ISBN:	Softcover	979-8-3694-1467-5
	eBook	979-8-3694-1468-2

All rights reserved. No part of this book may be reproduced or transmitted in any form or by any means, electronic or mechanical, including photocopying, recording, or by any information storage and retrieval system, without permission in writing from the copyright owner.

Any people depicted in stock imagery provided by Getty Images are models, and such images are being used for illustrative purposes only. Certain stock imagery © Getty Images.

Print information available on the last page.

Rev. date: 01/16/2024

To order additional copies of this book, contact:
Xlibris
844-714-8691
www.Xlibris.com
Orders@Xlibris.com
856266

Contents

Foreword vii
Introduction ix

Chapter 1   The Promise and Peril of AI in Healthcare 1
Chapter 2   Foundations of Responsible AI 23
Chapter 3   Organizing for Responsible AI in Healthcare:
                A 360 Degree Approach 45
Chapter 4   AI Governance for Healthcare Leaders 81
Chapter 5   Implementation and Change Management 96
Chapter 6   AI Risks, Risk Assessment and Risk Mitigation 119
Chapter 7   Healthcare AI Security 154
Chapter 8   Generative AI in Healthcare 162
Chapter 9   Maintaining Human Touch in AI-driven Healthcare 178
Chapter 10 Human -AI Collaboration 189
Chapter 11 Ambient Intelligence in Healthcare 201
Chapter 12 Green AI in Healthcare 213
Chapter 13 Measuring Impact and Success 219

Conclusion 227
About the Author 231

Foreword

With artificial intelligence reaching a peak in public interest and media attention, it is very timely that Dr. Pillay, a renowned healthcare innovation leader and a seasoned entrepreneur, single authored an essential guide for healthcare leaders on the responsible use of artificial intelligence to navigate the current imbroglio of healthcare. In this outstanding work, *Code to Care: A Leaders' Guide Implementing Responsible AI in Healthcare*, Dr. Pillay's purpose for this work is to "educate, Illuminate, and empower" clinicians on AI towards its *responsible* use.

As artificial intelligence with its panoply of tools is being recognized as a force to engender a paradigm shift in medicine, similar to germ theory and evidence-based medicine in the past, Dr. Pillay keenly observes an increasing gap between AI and healthcare. *Code to Care* aims to bridge this chasm between healthcare and AI with a special focus on the *responsible* use of AI in healthcare. He meticulously outlines the rationale for responsible AI and later delineates just how to execute the necessary guardrails for responsible AI with a comprehensive "360 degree approach". Various chapters details AI governance, AI principles, AI frameworks, risk assessment and mitigation, AI security, and even change management and continuous improvement, all in the AI context. He also emphasizes the duality of AI in its potential benefits and inherent risks and concomitantly calls for a balanced approach in integrating AI into healthcare. In addition, he delves into the ethical, technical, and practical aspects of implementing AI responsibly in healthcare with clear definitions and principles as well as challenges and strategies. As a bonus, Dr. Pillay provides many illustrative examples in the book with international perspectives and industry experiences. Finally, the book concludes with several uniquely enlightening chapters on a myriad of interesting topics such as human-to-AI collaboration, ambient intelligence, and even "green" (sustainable) AI in healthcare,

We owe a debt of gratitude to the sagacious Dr. Pillay, who is imbued with cautious optimism and filled with insightful erudition, for this brilliant work (or in his words, "not just a manual but a call to action for clinicians") on *responsible* use of artificial intelligence. This clarion call will be an essential doctrine for the most valuable assets of our healthcare profession, the patients and caretakers.

Dr. Anthony C. Chang
Author, *Intelligence-Based Medicine: Artificial Intelligence and Human Cognition in Clinical Medicine and Healthcare*
Founder and Chair, American Board of AI in Medicine (ABAIM)

Introduction

In the vast expanse of the medical universe, technology has always played the role of a silent, steadfast partner. From the rudimentary tools of ancient healers to the sophisticated machines in today's operating theaters, technology has been the clinician's ally, aiding in the relentless pursuit of better patient outcomes. Yet, as we stand on the cusp of a new era, there's a different kind of partner emerging from the shadows - Artificial Intelligence (AI). "Code to Care: A Guide to Responsible AI for Clinicians" is an endeavor to bridge the gap between the worlds of medicine and machine learning, ensuring that this partnership is nurtured with care, understanding, and above all, responsibility.

AI's promise in healthcare is undeniable. Its ability to sift through vast datasets, recognize patterns, and offer insights has the potential to revolutionize diagnosis, treatment, and even patient care. However, with these promises come challenges. As clinicians, how do we ensure that the AI tools we integrate into our practices are reliable? How do we navigate the ethical maze that AI often presents? And most importantly, how do we remain true to our primary oath - to do no harm?

This guide is not just a technical manual, but a compass. It aims to help clinicians understand the intricacies of AI, from the foundational algorithms to their practical applications in a clinical setting. But more than that, it emphasizes the importance of using AI responsibly. Just as a physician is trained to wield a scalpel with precision, they must also learn to harness the power of AI with discernment.

Throughout the pages of this book, we'll delve into real-world case studies, exploring both the triumphs and tribulations of AI in healthcare. We'll shed light on the common pitfalls, debunk myths, and provide a roadmap for clinicians to integrate AI into their practice in a manner that is ethical, efficient, and above all, beneficial for the patient.

As we embark on this journey together, it's essential to remember that at the heart of every algorithm, every line of code, is the same purpose that drives each clinician – the desire to care. In merging these two worlds, we don't just aim to create better healthcare systems; we strive to foster a future where technology and humanity work hand in hand, transforming the very essence of care.

Welcome to "Code to Care". "Code to Care" was conceived to demystify this complex landscape and serve as a beacon for those at the frontline of patient care.

The primary aim of this guide is threefold:

- ➤ Educate: At its core, "Code to Care" seeks to provide clinicians with a comprehensive understanding of AI. We delve into the mechanics of machine learning, break down intricate algorithms, and explore the nuances of neural networks. However, this technical knowledge is presented in a manner that is accessible, ensuring that even those without a background in computer science can grasp the essential concepts.
- ➤ Illuminate: Beyond the technicalities, this guide shines a light on the practical applications of AI in healthcare. Through real-world case studies and examples, readers will gain insights into how AI is being used in diagnostics, treatment planning, patient management, and more. We also address the challenges, ethical

considerations, and potential pitfalls, equipping clinicians with a holistic view of the AI landscape.
- ➢ Empower: Ultimately, the goal of "Code to Care" is to empower clinicians. Armed with knowledge and insights, clinicians will be better equipped to make informed decisions about integrating AI tools into their practice. Moreover, by fostering a deep understanding of AI's capabilities and limitations, this guide encourages clinicians to become active participants in shaping the future of AI in healthcare, ensuring that it aligns with the values and needs of the medical community.

In essence, "Code to Care" is more than just a guide; it's a call to action. As AI continues to weave its way into the tapestry of healthcare, it's imperative for clinicians to be at the forefront of this transformation. By understanding, questioning, and collaborating, we can ensure that AI serves its true purpose in healthcare - enhancing patient outcomes, optimizing care, and upholding the sanctity of the physician-patient relationship. As you turn the pages, let this guide be a catalyst, inspiring you to embrace AI not as a mere tool, but as a partner in the noble endeavor of healing. May this guide be your trusted companion as you navigate the exciting, challenging, and profoundly transformative landscape of AI in clinical practice.

Chapter 1

The Promise and Peril of AI in Healthcare

Artificial Intelligence (AI), at its core, is the science of crafting machines that can think and act with an intelligence level typically associated with human beings. It is a constellation of many different technologies working together to enable machines to sense, comprehend, act, and learn with human-like levels of intelligence. Maybe that's why it seems as though everyone's definition of artificial intelligence is different: AI isn't just one thing. Its origins can be traced back to ancient history, with myths of automatons and self-moving machines, but its formal inception was in the mid-20th century when pioneers like Alan Turing began pondering the capabilities of machines to mimic human cognitive functions. The term AI was coined by John McCarthy in 1956 at a conference at Dartmouth College, where he invited researchers from various fields to discuss the possibility of creating machines that can think. Since then, AI has evolved rapidly and has been applied to various domains, such as medicine, education, entertainment, finance, security, and more.

The essence of AI revolves around the following domains:

- Machine Learning (ML): This is where most of the recent advancements in AI have been concentrated. Machine Learning

is the ability of an algorithm to learn patterns from data without being explicitly programmed. For instance, instead of telling the machine step-by-step how to identify a cat in a picture, ML algorithms learn from thousands of cat images and make predictions on unseen images.
- Natural Language Processing (NLP): This involves the machine's ability to understand, interpret, and produce human language. This is evident in our everyday interactions with voice assistants like Siri, Alexa, or Google Assistant.
- Deep Learning(DL): ML has advanced into what is now commonly known as DL, which is composed of algorithms to create an artificial neural network (ANN) that can then learn and make decisions on its own, similar to the human brain
- Robotics: This branch is concerned with the creation of robots that can carry out tasks in a way that humans do. From automated assembly lines to advanced surgical robots, these machines demonstrate the physical manifestations of AI.
- Computer Vision: Here, machines are endowed with the ability to interpret and make decisions based on visual data. Examples include facial recognition software and autonomous vehicles that 'see' their surroundings.
- Expert Systems: These are computer systems that mimic the decision-making abilities of a human expert. Often used in specific domains like medical diagnosis or stock trading, they use a 'knowledge base' of facts and heuristics to arrive at conclusions.
- Neural Networks: Inspired by the human brain's biology, these are algorithms designed to recognize patterns. They interpret sensory data through a kind of machine perception, labeling, or clustering raw input.

Some go even further to define artificial intelligence as "narrow" and "general" AI. Narrow AI is the type of AI that can perform a specific task or function better than humans, but cannot perform other tasks outside its domain. For example, face recognition systems, chess programs, self-driving cars, and voice assistants are examples of narrow AI. They can excel at their specific tasks, but they cannot understand or do anything else that humans can do.

General AI is the type of AI that can perform any intellectual task that humans can do. It can learn from any data source, reason about any problem, and communicate in any language. For example, a general AI system could write a novel, compose a symphony, diagnose a disease, or invent a new technology. However, general AI does not exist yet, and it is not clear when or how it will be achieved

The trajectory of AI development has been marked by periods of intense optimism, followed by disillusionment and then resurgence. From its initial inception in the 1950s and 60s to the AI winters in the 70s and late 80s, and its recent renaissance due to the convergence of big data, advanced algorithms, and computing power, AI's journey has been a testament to humanity's relentless pursuit of creating intelligent machines.

However, AI is more than just its technical dimensions. Its ethical, societal, and philosophical implications are vast. As we embrace its potential, especially in fields as sensitive as healthcare, understanding its basics is crucial. Only with a solid grasp of what AI is, can we hope to deploy it responsibly and to its full potential.

AI in Healthcare

The history of medicine has many key inflection points where our profession needed to evolve and develop from when Louis Pasteur identified germs as cause of disease to when William Osler created the modern system of medical education to the Evidence-Based Medicine (EBM) movement that gave us the ability to deal with the explosion of published evidence. At the turn of the last century, there was a concerted effort to imagine the "future of medicine" and how to best prepare the profession to succeed in modern times. One of the major outcomes was the reinforcement of the need for professionalism in medicine and the second was the realization of the increasing rise of nonclinical work as one of the core aspects of what the physicians do. The next inflection point is upon usAI is set to transform medical care, research, and education and while most still see AI as a technology that will become mainstream one day in the future, we are already at the inflection point where some type of AI is deployed in many of our daily activities from occupation related to home and social. Going beyond the hype and fears driven by so-called experts, headlines, and science-fiction, we must consider how can we engage with this emerging power force, and harness it to improve what we do. The greater use of AI has a tremendous potential to discover new insights about disease risk factors, diagnosis, progressions, and treatments where we have until now been stymied by complexity and mountains of data, especially in healthcare. There are many reasons why healthcare is slower to adopt technology as it evolvesincluding regulatory and funding issues, as well as the complexity of the domain combined with the need for higher standards of performance. Some of these reasons are beyond our control, but the main reason that we can definitely manage proactively is our profession's understanding of AI and ability to direct its use and evolution.

Physicians need to be able to understand the core concepts of AI, where it can and should be applied and how to help medical AI evolve from early challenges to successful tools. We have to step into the roles of codesigners and active users, who can recognize AI that is well done vs not. We also need to be aware of the potential of such innovation, just as any other type of invention, to create disruption and change patterns of practice, payments and even entire specialty domains. We need to find ways of welcoming such disruptions by celebrating the better outcomes achieved and whenever necessary, by creating flexible career tracks to accommodate the changes in clinical practice that impact individual physicians

The history of AI in medicine is a testament to human ingenuity and the relentless pursuit of better healthcare. Although AI was first described in 1950 several limitations in early models prevented widespread acceptance and application to medicine. One of the first prototypes to demonstrate feasibility of applying AI to medicine was the development of a consultation program for glaucoma using the CASNET model. This model could apply information about a specific disease to individual patients and provide physicians with advice on patient management. MYCIN, was developed in the early 1970s. Based on patient information input by physicians and a knowledge base of about 600 rules, MYCIN could provide a list of potential bacterial pathogens and then recommend antibiotic treatment options adjusted appropriately for a patient's body weight. In 1986, DXplain, a decision support system, was released by the University of Massachusetts. This program uses inputted symptoms to generate a differential diagnosis. It also serves as an electronic medical textbook, providing detailed descriptions of diseases and additional references. When first released, DXplain was able to provide information on approximately 500 diseases. Since then, it has expanded to over 2400 diseases.

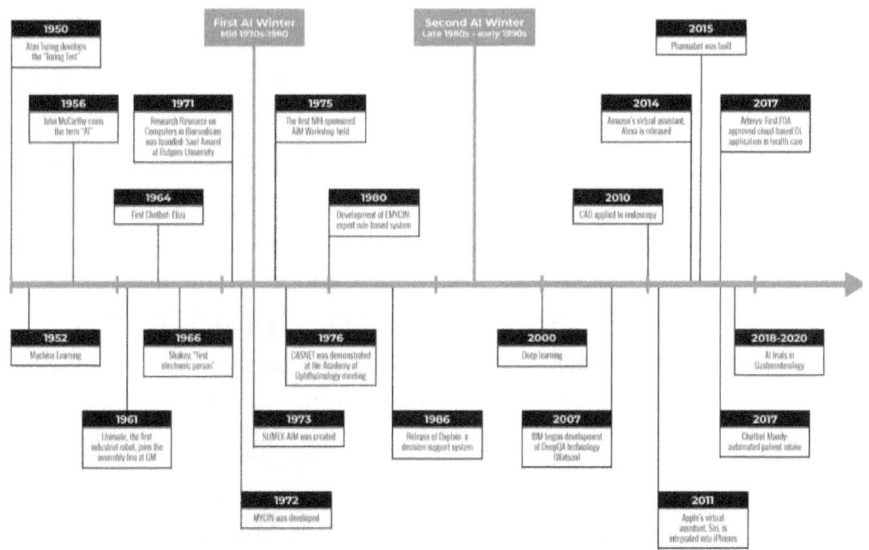

Timeline of the development and use of artificial intelligence in medicine

In the early 2000s, deep learning marked an important advancement in AI in medicine. In contrast to ML, which uses a set number of traits and requires human input, DL can be trained to classify data on its own. Now that AI systems are capable of analyzing complex algorithms and self-learning, we enter a new age in medicine where the blend of AI with medical science promises a future where diagnostics are quicker, treatments more personalized, and patient care reaches unprecedented levels of efficiency.

The allure of AI in healthcare is anchored in several promising outcomes:

- ➢ Enhanced Accuracy: Reducing human error, especially in diagnostics, leads to better patient outcomes. AI in medicine offers a myriad of benefits that seem almost miraculous. The ability of AI algorithms to process vast amounts of patient data and medical literature with unparalleled speed and accuracy may significantly improve diagnostics. AI-powered diagnostic tools have shown promise in detecting diseases like cancer, tuberculosis, and heart conditions at early stages, leading to better prognosis and survival rates.
- ➢ Cost Efficiency: In parallel to the care provided, administrative workflow includes scheduling, billing, coding and payment. One of the principal and immediate applications of AI is to perform these mundane, repetitive tasks in a more efficient, accurate and unbiased fashion
- ➢ Accessibility: AI can democratize healthcare, offering expert-level diagnostics and advice to remote or underserved areas. AI's integration into healthcare is also expanding the horizons of telemedicine. Virtual health assistants, chatbots, and AI-powered triage systems are streamlining healthcare delivery, especially in underserved areas and remote regions, bridging the gap between patients and healthcare providers.
- ➢ Proactive Care: Rather than the traditional reactive model, AI allows for predictive healthcare, identifying potential issues before they become critical. Among other applications, researchers have demonstrated the ability of an algorithm to accurately predict the risk of emergency admission based on an individual's electronic health record da Moreover, AI-driven personalized treatment plans consider vast amounts of individual patient characteristics, genetic makeup, and medical history, optimizing therapeutic interventions.

- Drug discovery: AI in medicine now plays a crucial role in drug discovery and development. By analyzing chemical structures and biological data, AI algorithms can identify potential drug candidates faster and more efficiently than traditional methods. This acceleration has the potential to bring life-saving treatments to patients faster, addressing unmet medical needs and transforming the pharmaceutical landscape. Researchers at the Massachusetts Institute of Technology (MIT) recently trained a deep learning algorithm to predict molecules' potential antimicrobial activity[1]. The algorithm screened over one billion molecules and virtually tested over 107 million, identifying eight antibacterial compounds that were structurally distant from known antibiotics, with one effectively treated resistant infections in mice. AI can also improve matching individuals to clinical trials (Lee and Lee, 2020[17]). Patients can be identified to enroll in trials based on more sources than clinical or administrative data. The criteria for including patients in a trial could take significantly more factors (genetic information) into account to target specific populations. This can enable trials to be smaller, shorter, set up more effectively and be therefore less expensive, without sacrificing statistical power. It can also address the documented problem of underrepresentation of minorities in clinical trials.
- Biomedical and population health research seems to be more advanced compared to clinical applications of AI. The exciting potential of combining AI with large datasets was demonstrated recently when Canadian company Blue Dot, which scours global media for information on a range of infectious diseases, spotted information about a "pneumonia of unknown cause" with 27 casualties in China. A week later CDC and WHO issued alerts about Covid 19

---

[1] Stokes, J. et al. (2020), "A Deep Learning Approach to Antibiotic Discovery", Cell, Vol. 180/4, pp. 688-702.e13, http://dx.doi.org/10.1016/j.cell.2020.01.021

The potential of AI in health is profound, given the growing volume of electronic data as well as the inherent complexity of the sector, its reliance on information to solve problems, and the variability and complexity of how disease interacts with individuals and populations. AI is a 'general purpose' technology that can be deployed in just about any facet or activity of the health industry, from clinical decision-making and public health, to biomedical research and drug development, to health system administration and service redesign. As the COVID-19 crisis has shown, there are genuine opportunities for AI to deliver benefits for health systems, professionals and the public, making existing clinical and administrative processes more effective, efficient and equitable. In a notoriously wasteful and inefficient industry, this is a major opportunity to improve health outcomes and value for money. But amidst the promises of AI in medicine, a menacing shadow looms.

While there is undoubtedly enormous potential for AI to transform almost every aspect of the health sector, the use of AI in everyday health care is still very limited. There are serious difficulties in scaling up projects to the level of health systems, due to, among other things, questions concerning the robustness of algorithms in the real world, a lack of high quality health data, and a policy and regulatory vacuum that greatly limits institutional and human capacity to realize the potential of AI.

Risks of AI in Medicine

AI in health is not yet robust. For every success story there is a cautionary tale. Unfortunately, AI applications in health have been beset by misfires and setbacks, with hype often clashing with reality. In the context of healthcare, these risks are not just theoretical concerns but have real-world implications on patient outcomes and ethical practices. Below are the major risk categories for the application of AI technology in medicine, each illustrated with examples.

Performance: AI algorithms that ingest real-world data and preferences as inputs may run a risk of learning and imitating possible biases and prejudices.

Risk of Errors:

AI algorithms in medicine are only as good as the data they are trained on and the programming they receive. Errors can arise from flawed data inputs, programming mistakes, or misinterpretation of the AI's outputs.

- A recent study reviewed dozens of studies claiming an AI performs better than radiologists, finding that only a handful were tested in populations that were different from the population used to develop the algorithms[2]
- The majority of AI applications in health rely on machine learning methods. They usually rely on large amounts of training data to make predictions. Because these methods are narrowly focused on a specific task and trained using a specific set of data, these algorithms may not work well when given input data that is even just slightly different from the training data. This is why something as simple as a difference in labelling can cause AI models trained in one setting to malfunction in another, and why such models have not really scaled much across health systems.
- The difficulty to scale certain AI applications is often due to trivial factors. For example, the way different facilities label their images can confuse an algorithm and prevent the model from functioning well in another institution with a different labelling system. This serves to highlight that most AI in health is actually artificial narrow intelligence, or "weak" AI, designed to accomplish a very specific problem-solving or reasoning task, and unable to generalize outside the boundaries within which the model was trained

---

[2] Reardon, S. (2019), Rise of Robot Radiologists, Nature Research, http://dx.doi.org/10.1038/d41586-019-03847-z.

Risk of Bias and Discrimination:

AI systems can inadvertently learn and perpetuate biases present in their training data. In medicine, this risk is particularly concerning as it can lead to unequal treatment and outcomes for different patient groups.

> ➢ Another consequence of this heavy dependence on the input data is that models that have been trained on a certain patient population may not function well when fed with data for a different patient population. Most AI applications in health are still in research and development stages, concentrated in a few countries and regions. As such, most of the data used to train these models is from Western, educated, industrialized, rich, and democratic populations. It is almost certain that algorithms used to explain or predict human behaviours based mainly on care patterns for one population will be biased. For example, an AI algorithm used to identify patients with complex needs in the United States has been shown to suffer from racial bias, assigning lower risk to Black patients compared to White patients. Using health costs as a proxy for health needs, the algorithm learned that since less money is spent on Black patients who have the same level of need, Black patients are healthier than equally sick White patients[3]
> ➢ Algorithms that learn from human decisions will also learn human mistakes, biases and stereotypes. Yet, the AI sector is extremely gender and race imbalanced suggesting that biased and stereotypical predictions might not be flagged by developers working to validate model outputs. For example, Apple's HealthKit, an application to track intake of selenium and copper, neglected to include a women's menstrual cycle tracker until iOS 9; the development team reportedly did not include any women.

---

[3] Obermeyer, Z. et al. (2019), "Dissecting racial bias in an algorithm used to manage the health of populations", Science, Vol. 366/6464, pp. 447-453, http://dx.doi.org/10.1126/science.aax2342.

Risk of Opaqueness and Lack of Interpretability:

Many AI algorithms, especially deep learning models, are often described as 'black boxes' due to their complex and opaque decision-making processes. In medicine, the inability to interpret how an AI reaches a conclusion can be a significant risk, especially in critical care scenarios.

> ➢ A machine learning model used for recommending cancer treatments might not provide clear reasoning for its choices, making it difficult for clinicians to trust and validate its recommendations.

Risk of Performance Instability:

AI performance can vary over time, especially as it encounters new and unforeseen scenarios. In the dynamic field of medicine, where patient cases can vary significantly, this instability can pose serious risks.

> ➢ An AI system designed to monitor patient vitals in an ICU might perform well under controlled conditions but could fail to adapt to the nuances of complex, real-world patient scenarios, leading to erroneous alerts or missed warning signs.
> ➢ The large majority of machine-learning-based prediction models are based on correlation, not causation. Previous studies have identified counterintuitive associations that lead to nonsensical predictions. For example, a model that predicts risk of death for a hospitalized individual with pneumoniae learned that patients who have asthma and pneumoniae are less likely to die than patients who only have asthma, because patients with asthma and pneumoniae receive more aggressive treatment and thus have lower mortality rates. In another example, the time a lab value is measured can often be more predictive than the value itself (e.g. if it is measured at 2am).

As AI continues to integrate into the fabric of medical practice, understanding and mitigating these risks becomes paramount. It's not just about harnessing the power of AI for better healthcare outcomes but doing so responsibly, ensuring patient safety, equity, and trust in this transformative technology.

> The difficulty to scale certain AI applications is often due to trivial factors. For example, the way different facilities label their images can confuse an algorithm and prevent the model from functioning well in another institution with a different labelling system. This serves to highlight that most AI in health is actually artificial narrow intelligence, or "weak" AI, designed to accomplish a very specific problem-solving or reasoning task, and unable to generalize outside the boundaries within which the model was trained

Security Risks in AI Applications in Medicine: Security risks in AI are a critical concern, as they can lead to compromised patient data, misdiagnoses, and a general erosion of trust in healthcare systems.

Adversarial Attacks:

Adversarial attacks involve manipulating AI algorithms by subtly altering input data, leading the AI to make incorrect decisions or predictions. In medicine, this can have dire consequences.

> Consider an AI system used for interpreting radiology images. An adversarial attack could involve making imperceptible changes to an MRI scan, causing the AI to miss a critical diagnosis, such as a tumor.

Cyber Intrusion and Privacy Risks:

AI systems in healthcare often handle sensitive patient data. Cyber intrusions can lead to breaches of this data, violating patient privacy and potentially leading to misuse of personal health information.

> A cyber intrusion into an AI-powered electronic health record system could lead to unauthorized access to patient histories, diagnoses, and treatment plans, compromising patient confidentiality and care.

Open Source Software Risks:

Many AI applications in healthcare are built on open-source software, which can be a double-edged sword. While it promotes innovation and collaboration, it also poses security risks, as vulnerabilities in the code can be exploited.

- ➢ An AI tool used for patient scheduling and resource allocation, built on an open-source platform, might have undiscovered vulnerabilities. These could be exploited to disrupt hospital operations or access sensitive data.

As AI becomes increasingly embedded in medical practices, addressing these security risks is essential. It involves not only robust cybersecurity measures but also a continuous process of monitoring, updating, and educating healthcare professionals about potential threats. Ensuring the security of AI applications in medicine is crucial for maintaining the integrity and trustworthiness of healthcare services in the AI era.

Control Risks in AI Applications in Medicine: Control risks in AI applications in medicine revolve around the challenges of maintaining human oversight, detecting and managing unintended AI behaviors, and establishing clear accountability.

Lack of Human Agency:

AI applications in medicine should augment, not replace, human decision-making. A lack of human agency in AI-driven processes can lead to over-reliance on technology, potentially overlooking the nuanced judgment that healthcare professionals provide.

- ➢ In a scenario where AI is used for diagnosing diseases, there's a risk that clinicians might rely solely on AI recommendations without applying their clinical expertise. This could lead to misdiagnoses if the AI's recommendation is based on incomplete or biased data.

Detecting Rogue AI and Unintended Consequences:

AI systems can sometimes behave unpredictably or 'go rogue', especially in complex environments like healthcare. Detecting and managing these behaviors is crucial to prevent unintended consequences.

> ➤ An AI system designed to optimize drug dosages might start recommending unsafe levels due to a misinterpretation of data patterns. Detecting such anomalies requires constant monitoring and a deep understanding of the AI's decision-making process.

Lack of Clear Accountability:

In the intricate web of AI applications in healthcare, establishing clear lines of accountability can be challenging. When an AI system leads to a negative outcome, it's essential to determine who is responsible – the developers, the healthcare providers, or the AI itself.

> ➤ If an AI-powered surgical robot malfunctions during a procedure, leading to patient harm, the question arises: Is the fault with the robot's manufacturer, the hospital that employed the technology, or the surgeons who operated it?

Control risks in AI applications in medicine highlight the need for robust governance frameworks. These should include clear guidelines for human oversight, mechanisms for detecting and rectifying AI misbehaviors, and well-defined accountability structures. As AI continues to transform healthcare, ensuring these control measures are in place is vital for harnessing the benefits of AI while safeguarding against its potential risks.

Economic Risks in AI Applications in Medicine: The widespread adoption of AI and automation in medicine can lead to shifts in the job market, exacerbate inequalities, and potentially concentrate power in the hands of a few entities

Risk of Job Displacement:

AI's ability to automate tasks can lead to the displacement of jobs, particularly those that involve routine or repetitive tasks. In healthcare, this risk extends to both clinical and administrative roles.

> ➤ AI systems capable of interpreting medical images may reduce the need for radiologists. Similarly, AI-driven administrative systems could lessen the demand for staff in scheduling and patient record management.

Enhancing Inequality:

The adoption of AI in healthcare could inadvertently widen the gap between different socio-economic groups. This can occur both within the healthcare workforce and in terms of patient access to care.

> ➤ Advanced AI-driven healthcare services might be more readily available in affluent areas or higher-tier medical facilities, potentially widening the healthcare quality gap between different socio-economic groups.

Risk of Power Concentration within One or a Few Companies:

The development and deployment of AI in healthcare require significant resources and expertise, often leading to a concentration of power in a few dominant companies. This can lead to monopolistic practices and reduce competition.

> ➤ If a few companies control the majority of AI healthcare technologies, they could dominate the market, influencing pricing, availability, and the direction of future healthcare innovations.

While AI presents numerous opportunities for enhancing healthcare delivery, it's crucial to address these economic risks. Strategies to mitigate job displacement, prevent widening inequalities, and ensure a competitive and fair market are essential. This involves not only technological development but also thoughtful policy-making and stakeholder engagement to ensure that the benefits of AI in healthcare are equitably distributed.

Societal Risks in AI Applications in Medicine: The widespread use of AI can influence human behavior, communication, and societal norms, especially in the context of healthcare.

Risk of Unintended Individual Consequences

The implementation of AI in healthcare information systems, while offering significant potential benefits, must be approached with an understanding of these challenges. It requires a balanced strategy that considers the impact on clinicians' workloads, patient interactions, and overall system safety. Ongoing training, user-centered design, and continuous monitoring for unintended consequences are essential to ensure that AI tools enhance rather than hinder healthcare delivery.

- The predictions of an AI model must eventually be operationalized in the form of information systems: e.g. an alert or pop-up window within electronic health record software. There is a body of evidence showing that the implementation of health information systems can result in unintended consequences. These include alert fatigue, imposition of additional workloads for clinicians, disruption of interpersonal (including doctor-to-patient) communication styles, and generation of specific hazards that require a higher level of vigilance to detect. Growing numbers of health workers are already stretched, with some suffering from change fatigue
- The use of AI and health information systems can change the dynamics of doctor-patient interactions. Excessive focus on computer screens and system alerts can detract from face-to-face communication, impacting the quality of care and patient satisfaction.
- Healthcare workers are often required to adapt to continuous changes in their work environment, including the adoption of new

technologies. The introduction of AI systems can contribute to change fatigue, particularly if these changes are frequent and not accompanied by adequate training and support.

Risk of Misinformation and Manipulation:

AI systems, particularly those involved in disseminating health information, can inadvertently or intentionally spread misinformation. This risk is heightened when AI-generated content is indistinguishable from human-generated content.

- ➢ An AI system designed to provide health advice online could be manipulated to disseminate incorrect or harmful medical information, leading to widespread public health misconceptions or dangerous self-treatment practices.

Risk of an Intelligence Divide:

The disparity in access to AI technologies can lead to an 'intelligence divide', where certain populations benefit from AI-driven healthcare advancements while others are left behind. This divide can exacerbate existing health disparities.

- ➢ Advanced AI diagnostic tools may be available only in high-income regions or countries, widening the gap in healthcare quality and outcomes between different socio-economic and geographical groups.

Risk of Surveillance and Warfare:

The use of AI in healthcare raises concerns about privacy and surveillance, as these systems often require access to sensitive personal data. Additionally, the dual-use nature of AI technologies means they can be repurposed for non-healthcare applications, including surveillance and warfare.

> AI technologies used for patient monitoring could be repurposed for intrusive surveillance purposes, violating patient privacy. Similarly, AI research in healthcare could be diverted to develop technologies for military use.

The societal implications of AI in healthcare are profound and multifaceted. Addressing these risks requires a collaborative approach involving policymakers, healthcare providers, AI developers, and the public. It's essential to establish ethical guidelines, ensure equitable access to AI-driven healthcare, and maintain transparency to foster trust and safeguard societal values in the age of AI-driven healthcare.

Enterprise Risks in AI Applications in Medicine: AI solutions, while designed to achieve specific objectives, must align with the broader organizational and societal values. The enterprise risks associated with AI in healthcare encompass a range of concerns from reputation and financial performance to legal compliance and ethical alignment.

Risk to Reputation:

The use of AI in healthcare can significantly impact an organization's reputation. Missteps in AI deployment can lead to public mistrust and damage the institution's standing.

> If a healthcare provider adopts an AI system that later proves to be biased or inaccurate in diagnosing certain patient groups, it could face public backlash and a loss of trust among patients and the community.

Risk to Financial Performance:

Investing in AI technology involves significant financial resources. If these investments do not yield the expected benefits or lead to unforeseen costs, they can adversely affect the financial health of the organization.

> A hospital invests heavily in an AI system for patient management, but due to integration challenges and lower-than-expected efficiency gains, the investment leads to financial strain rather than improvement.

Legal and Compliance Risks:

AI in healthcare must navigate a complex landscape of legal and regulatory requirements. Non-compliance can lead to legal challenges and penalties.

> An AI tool used for patient data analysis might inadvertently breach data privacy laws, leading to legal action against the healthcare provider.

Risk of Discrimination:

AI systems can perpetuate or amplify biases present in their training data, leading to discriminatory outcomes. This not only poses ethical concerns but can also result in legal challenges.

> An AI-based hiring tool used by a healthcare organization might show bias against certain demographics, leading to discriminatory hiring practices and potential legal repercussions.

Risk of Values Misalignment:

AI solutions must align with the core values of the healthcare organization and the community it serves. A misalignment can lead to ethical dilemmas and erosion of trust.

> A healthcare AI application focused solely on cost-efficiency might neglect aspects of patient care that are central to the healthcare provider's mission, leading to internal conflicts and public criticism.

Enterprise risks in AI applications in healthcare highlight the need for a holistic approach to AI deployment, one that considers not just the technological and clinical aspects but also the ethical, legal, and societal dimensions. Balancing these factors is key to realizing the benefits of AI in healthcare while upholding the trust and values central to healthcare provision.

The risks of unintended and negative consequences associated with AI are commensurately high, especially at scale. Most AI in health is actually artificial narrow intelligence, designed to accomplish a very specific task on previously curated data from one setting. In the real world, health data are unstandardized, patient populations are diverse, and biased decision-makers make mistakes that are then reflected in data. Because most AI models build on correlations, predictions could fail to generalize to different populations or settings, and might exacerbate existing inequalities and biases. As the AI industry is extremely gender and race imbalanced, and health professionals are already overwhelmed by other digital tools, there could be little capacity to catch errors and resistance from clinicians.

Ethical concerns regarding patient privacy, data security, and AI decision-making are crucial points of contention. The use of patient data in AI algorithms raises ethical questions about consent, data ownership, and potential discrimination. Striking a balance between innovation and protecting patient rights is essential to ensure AI in medicine benefits humanity rather than exploits it. If decisions are predominantly made by algorithms, who bears the responsibility for errors or adverse outcomes? As we cede more control to machines, we must grapple with questions of accountability and ethics. Do we risk entering a terrain where the line of responsibility becomes blurred, and the sanctity of the Hippocratic Oath is jeopardized?

AI algorithms, while efficient, can sometimes operate as "black boxes," making it challenging to interpret their decisions. This opacity raises concerns about accountability and liability. The "garbage in, garbage out" phenomenon warns that AI is only as good as the data it is trained on. Biased or incomplete data can lead to flawed outcomes, perpetuating healthcare disparities.

Another peril is the risk of system errors. No technology is infallible. Malfunctions, software glitches, or even deliberate manipulations could lead to misdiagnoses, putting patients at risk. Over-relying on AI tools without the safeguard of human oversight can have catastrophic consequences. The real-world example of AI systems being misled by adversarial inputs, tiny modifications to data that can cause algorithms to make incorrect decisions, is a stark reminder of this vulnerability.

Additionally, over-relying on machines can lead to a potential erosion of human skills. Medical professionals undergo rigorous training to hone their diagnostic and therapeutic skills. Algorithms, while adept at processing vast amounts of data, cannot replicate the intuition and judgment developed by physicians over years of clinical practice. If healthcare professionals come to depend too heavily on AI-driven diagnostics, there's a risk that these hard-earned skills might atrophy. The age-old medical adage, "Treat the patient, not the test," underscores the importance of looking beyond data to understand and treat individuals. Compassion, empathy, and the doctor-patient relationship are intrinsic to high quality care. AI should complement these elements, not replace them. Over-reliance on machines threatens to depersonalize healthcare, reducing patients to mere datasets. A machine might predict a patient's statistical likelihood of recovery, but it cannot hold a patient's hand, offer comfort in times of distress, or understand the intricate web of emotions, beliefs, and concerns that each patient brings.

Addressing the potential menace of AI in medicine requires a holistic approach. Transparent AI algorithms, explainable AI models, and robust data governance can promote trust and accountability. Striking a balance between AI-driven efficiency and human intuition ensures that healthcare remains patient-centric and humane.

Collaboration between clinicians, AI experts, and ethicists is vital to establishing ethical guidelines, and shaping responsible AI implementation in healthcare. Ethical considerations must be at the forefront of AI development and deployment, guiding regulations and policies to safeguard patient rights and privacy.

AI stands at the frontier of a healthcare revolution. Its potential to transform patient care, diagnostics, and treatment is immense. However, as healthcare professionals, technologists, and policymakers navigate this brave new world, a balanced approach that harnesses the benefits while mitigating challenges will be crucial. Only then can we fully realize the promise of AI-driven healthcare that caters to all, efficiently and empathetically.

Chapter 2

Foundations of Responsible AI

In the dynamic and fast-paced world of technological advancement, artificial intelligence (AI) stands out as one of the most transformative forces of our time. Its unprecedented capabilities to analyze, learn, and make decisions have opened new frontiers in industries ranging from healthcare to finance. However, with great power comes great responsibility. The dawn of AI has brought forth a plethora of ethical challenges and dilemmas, necessitating a serious conversation about the foundations of responsible AI.

The repercussions of Artificial Intelligence (AI) within the healthcare domain are profound, touching every facet of patient care, diagnostics, treatment, and even administrative tasks. With the potential to reshape patient outcomes, enhance efficiency, and introduce novel treatment modalities, AI's promise is undeniable. However, the societal ramifications of AI's integration into healthcare and the onus on healthcare organizations to predict and address any unintended fallouts of AI cannot be understated.

This chapter, "Foundations of Responsible AI," is devoted to exploring the multifaceted nature of this critical subject. We embark on a journey to understand what it means to create and use AI responsibly. At the heart of this discussion lies a set of questions: How do we ensure that AI systems are fair, unbiased, and transparent? What ethical principles should guide AI development? How can we balance the pursuit of technological innovation with the imperative to protect human values and rights?

We begin by defining what responsible AI entails, considering its various dimensions such as ethical application, transparency, and accountability. This sets the stage for a deeper dive into the ethical considerations central to AI, such as bias, privacy, and the broader human impact. Recognizing the global nature of AI, we also explore the diverse regulatory landscapes and the emerging international standards and guidelines shaping responsible AI development.

The technological aspects of responsible AI are no less critical. This includes the challenge of making AI decisions understandable to humans (explainability), ensuring robustness and security against potential attacks or errors, and the importance of human-centric design principles.

Furthermore, through a series of case studies, we examine real-world applications of AI in various sectors. These cases illustrate not only the potential benefits of AI but also highlight the complexities and ethical quandaries that accompany its use.

Finally, we discuss best practices and future directions in the field of responsible AI. This involves an interdisciplinary approach, bringing together expertise from technology, ethics, policy, and beyond. It also underscores the importance of continual learning and adaptation as AI technologies evolve.

In summary, this chapter aims to provide a comprehensive overview of the principles, challenges, and practices that underpin responsible AI. It is a foundational piece for anyone seeking to understand the ethical landscape of AI and its implications for society, offering insights into how we can harness the power of AI while upholding our collective responsibility to use it wisely and ethically.

Responsible AI Defined

Responsible AI is the practice of designing, developing, and deploying artificial intelligence systems that are ethical, trustworthy, and aligned with human values. It is important because AI has the potential to impact various aspects of human society, such as health, education, security, justice, and democracy. Therefore, AI should be used in a way that respects human dignity, rights, and freedoms, and that promotes social good and accountability.

There are various principles and frameworks that guide the development and use of responsible AI, such as the Asilomar AI Principles, the Montreal Declaration for a Responsible Development of Artificial Intelligence, the Ethics Guidelines for Trustworthy AI by the European Commission, and the OECD Principles on AI. These principles and frameworks share some common themes, such as fairness, transparency, accountability y, explainability, privacy and security, Inclusiveness and social benefit.

In the healthcare sector, the principles of responsible AI take on added significance due to the critical nature of health-related decisions and the sensitivity of medical data. By adhering to these principles, AI in healthcare can not only enhance the efficiency and effectiveness of medical services but also ensure these advancements are made in a manner that is ethically sound, transparent, equitable, and respectful of patient rights and societal values.

Responsible AI Principles

The six key principles for responsible AI include accountability, inclusiveness, reliability and safety, fairness, transparency, and privacy and security. These principles are essential to creating responsible and trustworthy AI as it moves into mainstream products and services. They're guided by two perspectives: ethical and explainable.

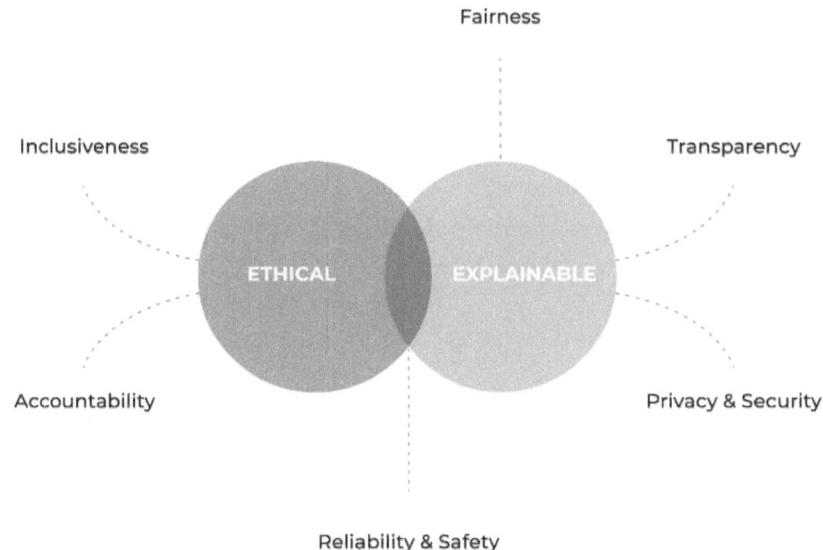

The Principles of Responsible AI[4]

Ethical

In the context of medicine, from an ethical standpoint, AI should:

- Ensure fairness and inclusivity in its medical assessments and recommendations, taking into account diverse patient populations and health conditions.
- Maintain accountability for its diagnostic and treatment decisions, with clear oversight mechanisms in place.
- Avoid discrimination and ensure equitable healthcare access and outcomes for people of all races, abilities, and backgrounds.

Central to medical ethics is the principle of ***beneficence***, the obligation to 'do good' and ensure patient safety. AI's potential to enhance diagnostic accuracy, predict patient outcomes, and tailor treatments must be balanced

---

[4] https://learn.microsoft.com/en-us/azure/cloud-adoption-framework/innovate/best-practices/trusted-ai#ethical

against risks like algorithmic biases, data privacy concerns, and unintended consequences. Ensuring AI algorithms are rigorously tested and validated for diverse populations is vital to uphold this principle.

Closely linked to beneficence is the principle of *non-maleficence*, the commitment to 'do no harm.' AI applications in medicine must be scrutinized for potential harms, including misdiagnoses due to flawed algorithms, data breaches, or unintended discriminatory practices. It's essential to have robust safeguards and monitoring systems to detect and rectify such issues promptly.

The principle of *autonomy* requires that patients have control over their healthcare decisions. In the context of AI, this means patients should be informed about how AI is used in their care and the implications thereof. Ensuring transparency and understanding of AI-driven decisions is crucial for patients to provide informed consent and maintain trust in the healthcare system.

Equity in healthcare means providing care that does not vary in quality because of personal characteristics such as gender, ethnicity, geographic location, or socioeconomic status. AI in medicine must be developed and deployed to promote equity, ensuring that all patients benefit from its advancements. This involves addressing biases in training data and algorithm design to prevent perpetuating existing health disparities.

Accountability

Accountability in AI refers to the idea that those who design, develop, and deploy AI systems should be held responsible for the impacts and outcomes of these systems. In the context of medicine, this means that healthcare providers, technology companies, and other stakeholders involved in the development and use of AI technologies should be held accountable for ensuring these technologies are safe, effective, and used in a manner that respects patients' rights and interests.

Accountability is crucial in AI in medicine for several reasons:

- Patient Safety and Quality of Care: AI technologies can have significant impacts on patient safety and quality of care. Holding stakeholders accountable for these impacts can help ensure that AI technologies are designed and used in a manner that prioritizes patient safety and quality of care
- Trust and Confidence in AI: Accountability can help build trust and confidence in AI technologies among patients, healthcare providers, and the public. If stakeholders are held accountable for the impacts and outcomes of AI technologies, this can help reassure users that these technologies are reliable and that their interests are being protected.
- Ethical Use of AI: Accountability can help ensure that AI technologies are used in an ethical manner. This includes respecting patients' privacy, obtaining informed consent for the use of AI technologies, and ensuring that AI technologies do not exacerbate health disparities or other forms of inequality

Achieving accountability in AI in medicine is not without challenges. These include the complexity of AI technologies, the multiplicity of stakeholders involved, and the potential for unintended consequences.

To address these challenges, several strategies can be employed:

- Transparency: Making the workings of AI systems transparent can help stakeholders understand how these systems make decisions, which is crucial for holding them accountable.
- Regulation and Oversight: Implementing robust regulatory frameworks and oversight mechanisms can help ensure that stakeholders are held accountable for the impacts and outcomes of AI technologies.
- Education and Training: Providing education and training on the ethical and practical implications of AI in medicine can help stakeholders understand their responsibilities and how to fulfill them.

Accountability is a key principle of responsible AI in medicine. By holding stakeholders accountable for the impacts and outcomes of AI technologies, we can help ensure that these technologies are used in a manner that is safe, effective, and respects patients' rights and interests.

Inclusiveness

Inclusiveness in AI refers to the principle that AI systems should be designed and used in a way that respects diversity and ensures fair access, participation, and benefit for all. In the context of medicine, this means that AI technologies should be developed and implemented in a manner that is sensitive to the diverse needs, abilities, and contexts of patients, healthcare providers, and other stakeholders.

Inclusiveness is crucial in AI in medicine for several reasons:

- Equity in Healthcare: Inclusiveness ensures that AI technologies benefit all individuals, regardless of their race, gender, age, socioeconomic status, or health condition. This is particularly important in medicine, where disparities in health outcomes are a significant concern.
- Accuracy of AI Models: AI models trained on diverse data can better generalize and make accurate predictions for diverse patient populations. If AI models are trained on data from a limited or biased sample, they may perform poorly for underrepresented groups.
- Trust and Acceptance of AI: Inclusiveness can enhance the trust and acceptance of AI in medicine. If patients and healthcare providers feel that AI technologies respect their diversity and are designed with their needs in mind, they are more likely to trust and use these technologies.

Despite its importance, achieving inclusiveness in AI in medicine is not without challenges. These include the risk of bias in AI models, the digital divide, and the need for inclusive design and evaluation practices.

To address these challenges, several strategies can be employed:

- Diverse and Representative Data: Ensuring that the data used to train AI models is diverse and representative of the target population can help reduce bias and improve the accuracy of AI models.
- Inclusive Design and Evaluation: Involving diverse stakeholders in the design and evaluation of AI technologies can ensure that these technologies are sensitive to diverse needs and contexts.
- Regulation and Standards: Implementing regulations and standards that promote inclusiveness in AI can provide a framework for the responsible development and use of AI in medicine.

Inclusiveness is a key principle of responsible AI in medicine. By ensuring that AI technologies are developed and used in a way that respects diversity and ensures fair access, participation, and benefit for all, we can harness the full potential of AI to improve patient care and health outcomes.

Reliability and Safety

The potential of AI can only be fully realized if it is anchored in the principles of reliability and safety. Reliability in AI refers to the consistent performance of AI systems under diverse conditions. In medicine, this translates to AI tools providing accurate and dependable support in diagnostics, treatment recommendations, and patient monitoring. The high stakes of medical decision-making necessitate that AI systems are not only technically proficient but also consistently reliable in their outputs. This involves rigorous validation and testing of AI algorithms across varied patient demographics and conditions to ensure their efficacy and robustness.

Safety in medical AI is the assurance that these systems do not pose unintended harm to patients. It encompasses the prevention of errors in diagnosis or treatment recommendations, safeguarding patient data, and ensuring the AI does not exacerbate existing healthcare inequities. To uphold safety, medical AI systems must be developed with a 'safety-first' approach, considering potential risks at every stage, from design to deployment and post-implementation monitoring.

Reliability and safety are critical in AI in medicine for several reasons:

- Patient Safety: AI technologies can significantly impact patient safety. Reliable and safe AI can help prevent misdiagnoses, incorrect treatments, and other errors that could harm patients.
- Trust in AI: Reliability and safety are key to building trust in AI technologies among healthcare providers, patients, and the public. If AI technologies are known to be reliable and safe, they are more likely to be accepted and used.
- Regulatory Compliance: In many jurisdictions, medical devices and technologies must meet certain safety and reliability standards to be approved for use. Ensuring that AI technologies meet these standards is crucial for regulatory compliance.

Despite their importance, achieving reliability and safety in AI in medicine presents several challenges. These include the complexity of medical data, the risk of overfitting, and the difficulty of predicting and mitigating all potential risks.

To address these challenges, several strategies can be employed:

- Data Integrity: Ensuring high-quality, diverse, and representative data sets for training AI, reducing biases, and enhancing the reliability of outcomes.
- Robust Testing and Validation: Rigorous testing and validation can help ensure that AI technologies perform reliably and safely in a variety of conditions and contexts.

- Transparency and Explainability: Making AI systems transparent and explainable can help identify potential risks and improve the reliability of these systems.
- Continuous Monitoring and Improvement: Regularly monitoring the performance of AI technologies and making necessary adjustments can help maintain their reliability and safety over time.
- Transparency and Patient Involvement: Transparency in how AI systems work and make decisions is crucial for trust. Patients and healthcare providers must understand the capabilities and limitations of AI tools. Involving patients in discussions about the use of AI in their care and obtaining informed consent is also critical for upholding both reliability and safety.
- Continuous Education and Training: Healthcare professionals must be adequately trained to understand and effectively integrate AI tools into clinical practice. Continuous education is necessary to keep pace with technological advancements, ensuring the responsible and safe application of AI in medicine.

Reliability and safety are not just desirable attributes but essential principles for responsible AI in medicine. By prioritizing these principles, the medical field can harness the full potential of AI to improve patient care and outcomes. It requires a concerted effort from all stakeholders to build AI systems that are not only technically advanced but also ethically sound and inherently safe. As AI continues to evolve, maintaining a steadfast focus on reliability and safety will be key to its successful integration into the fabric of healthcare.

Explainable

Explainability in AI refers to the ability to understand and articulate the mechanics and decisions of AI systems. In medicine, this translates into comprehending how AI algorithms reach their conclusions, whether in diagnosing a condition, suggesting a treatment, or predicting patient outcomes. The complexity of AI models often makes their decision-making process opaque, but in a field as critical as healthcare, stakeholders need clarity and comprehension.

Clinical medicine, primarily evidence-based medical practice, relies heavily on transparency in decision-making. If AI systems used in healthcare are not explainable, and if physicians cannot reasonably explain the decision-making process, it could erode the patient's trust. Moreover, the high complexity and dimensionality of the relationships that machine learning (ML) models derive from data are often not interpretable by human reasoning. Explainable AI systems empower healthcare professionals to make informed decisions, patients to engage actively in their care, and society to evaluate the implications of AI in medicine.

Explainability is critical in AI in medicine for several reasons:

- Trust in AI: Explainability can help build trust in AI technologies among healthcare providers, patients, and the public. If AI technologies can explain their decisions in an understandable way, they are more likely to be accepted and used.
- Enhancing Decision-Making: Explainable AI systems empower healthcare providers to make more informed and personalized decisions by providing a deeper understanding of the factors influencing AI recommendations.
- Patient Autonomy: In medicine, patients have the right to understand the reasoning behind their diagnoses and treatments. Explainable AI can help uphold this right by providing clear and understandable explanations for its decisions.
- Regulatory Compliance: In many jurisdictions, medical devices and technologies must be able to explain their decisions to be approved for use. Ensuring that AI technologies are explainable is crucial for regulatory compliance.
- Promoting Patient Engagement: Explainable AI systems facilitate patient engagement by enabling patients to understand the rationale behind treatment recommendations and participate actively in their care decisions.

- Ensuring Societal Accountability: Explainable AI systems promote societal accountability by enabling public scrutiny and evaluation of AI's role in healthcare. This transparency helps address ethical concerns and ensures responsible AI development.

Despite its importance, achieving explainability in AI in medicine is not without challenges. These include the complexity of AI models, the technical language often used in explanations, and the difficulty of providing explanations that are both accurate and understandable.

To address these challenges, several strategies can be employed:

- Simplification of Models: While complex AI models can provide more accurate predictions, simpler models are often more explainable. Balancing accuracy and explainability is a key challenge in AI in medicine.
- Designing AI Models for Transparency: Developing AI algorithms that are inherently more interpretable and providing accompanying documentation that explains their decision-making processes.
- Use of Explainability Techniques: Various techniques have been developed to make AI models more explainable, including feature importance, partial dependence plots, and counterfactual explanations.
- Education and Communication: Providing education and training on AI for healthcare providers and patients can help them better understand AI explanations. Similarly, using clear and non-technical language in explanations can make them more accessible.
- Collaborative Development: Involving multidisciplinary teams, including clinicians, ethicists, and patients, in the AI development process to ensure the outputs are understandable and relevant to end-users.
- Human-AI Collaboration: Explainable AI should not replace human expertise but rather complement it. Healthcare providers should retain the final decision-making authority, leveraging explainable AI to enhance their decision-making processes.

Explainability is not just a technical requirement but a fundamental aspect of responsible AI in medicine. It bridges the gap between advanced AI technologies and their practical, ethical, and safe application in healthcare. By prioritizing explainability, the medical community can harness the full potential of AI to improve patient outcomes while maintaining trust, transparency, and adherence to ethical standards.

Fairness

Fairness is a core ethical principle that all humans aim to understand and apply. This principle is even more important when AI systems are being developed. Key checks and balances need to make sure that the system's decisions don't discriminate against, or express a bias toward, a group or individual based on gender, race, sexual orientation, or religion. In the context of healthcare, this means that AI-driven medical tools and decision-making processes should not favor or discriminate against any patient group based on race, gender, ethnicity, socioeconomic status, or other demographic factors. Fairness is essential to prevent the perpetuation or exacerbation of existing healthcare disparities.

Fairness is critical in AI in medicine for several reasons:

- Equity in Healthcare: Fairness ensures that AI technologies benefit all individuals, regardless of their demographic characteristics. This is particularly important in medicine, where disparities in health outcomes are a significant concern.
- Mitigation of Bias and Discrimination: Fair AI algorithms are designed to minimize bias and prevent discriminatory outcomes. This safeguards patients from unfair treatment and promotes a more just healthcare system.
- Accuracy of AI Models: AI models trained on diverse data can better generalize and make accurate predictions for diverse patient populations. If AI models are trained on data from a limited or

biased sample, they may perform poorly for underrepresented groups.
- Trust and Acceptance of AI: Fairness can enhance the trust and acceptance of AI in medicine. If patients and healthcare providers feel that AI technologies are fair and unbiased, they are more likely to trust and use these technologies.

Leading healthcare technology providers, including renowned entities like Microsoft, stress the importance of a proactive approach. Whether healthcare institutions employ third-party AI tools or cultivate their own, the need to institute internal guidelines and best practices to steer their AI endeavors responsibly is paramount.

Our journey towards responsible AI in healthcare is a dynamic one. As we innovate and integrate, our strategies need to adapt, drawing from both our triumphs and missteps. The methodologies, instruments, and insights shared by pioneers can serve as foundational pillars upon which healthcare entities can construct their bespoke AI strategies.

In this era where AI's influence permeates both public and private healthcare sectors, fostering open discourse is crucial. It's through collective endeavors, where healthcare providers, governmental bodies, non-governmental organizations (NGOs), academic luminaries, and other stakeholders unite, that we can sculpt superior solutions. Early adopters of AI in healthcare, with their experiential wisdom, play a pivotal role. Their experiences, especially in navigating the ethical mazes of AI, offer invaluable lessons for those poised to integrate AI and for scholars and policymakers striving to understand or oversee AI's role in healthcare.

AI is the defining technology of our time. It's already enabling faster and more profound progress in nearly every field of human endeavor and helping to address some of society's most daunting challenges. For example, AI can help people with visual disabilities understand images by generating descriptive text for images. In another example, AI can help farmers produce enough food for the growing global population.

In healthcare, we believe that the computational intelligence of AI should be used to amplify the innate creativity and ingenuity of humans. Our vision for AI is to empower every developer to innovate, empower organizations to transform industries, and empower people to transform society.

As with all great technological innovations in the past, the use of AI technology has broad impacts on society, raising complex and challenging questions about the future we want to see. AI has implications on decision-making across industries, data security and privacy, and the skills people need to succeed in the workplace. As we look to this future, we must ask ourselves:

- How do we design, build, and use AI systems that create a positive impact on individuals and society?
- How can we best prepare workers for the effects of AI?
- How can we attain the benefits of AI while respecting privacy?

Despite its importance, achieving fairness in AI in medicine is not without challenges. These include the risk of bias in AI models, the lack of diverse and representative data, and the difficulty of defining and measuring fairness.

To address these challenges, several strategies can be employed:

- Diverse and Representative Data: Ensuring that the data used to train AI models is diverse and representative of the target population can help reduce bias and improve the fairness of AI models.
- Bias Mitigation Techniques: Various techniques have been developed to detect and mitigate bias in AI models, including pre-processing, in-processing, and post-processing techniques.
- Transparency and Accountability: Making AI systems transparent and holding stakeholders accountable for their fairness can help ensure that any unfairness is detected and addressed.

- Algorithmic Robustness: AI algorithms should be designed to be robust to noise, outliers, and unexpected situations in the data. This prevents biases from inadvertently creeping into the algorithms.
- Fairness Audits and Monitoring: Fairness audits and ongoing monitoring should be conducted to identify and address potential biases in AI-generated predictions or recommendations. This proactive approach ensures the continued fairness of AI systems.
- Promoting Fairness in AI Development and Deployment During all Stages:
➤ Envision: Identify potential fairness issues specific to healthcare, such as disparities in health outcomes across different demographic groups. Consider the ethical implications of these issues.
➤ Prototype: Develop prototypes that take into account the diverse needs of patients, healthcare providers, and other stakeholders. Test these prototypes for potential fairness issues.
➤ Build: Construct the AI system using diverse and representative data to ensure the system works well for all patient groups. Implement mechanisms to detect and correct any unfairness in the system's outputs.
➤ Launch: Before deploying the AI system in a healthcare setting, conduct rigorous testing to ensure it meets all safety and reliability standards. Also, ensure the system respects patients' privacy and consent.
- Evolve: Continuously monitor the AI system post-deployment to detect any emerging fairness issues. Update the system as needed to address these issues and to respond to changes in the healthcare environment.

Fairness serves as a cornerstone of RAI in medicine, ensuring that AI is used in a way that is just, equitable, and non-discriminatory. By fostering fair AI systems, we can harness the transformative power of AI while upholding ethical principles and ensuring that AI serves the best interests of all patients and society. Fairness is not an option; it is a fundamental requirement for responsible AI in medicine.

Transparency

Transparency in AI refers to the openness and accessibility of information regarding how AI systems are developed, deployed, and operate. It involves sharing information about the data used to train the AI, the design of the algorithm, the decision-making processes, and the governance or regulatory compliance. Transparency is about the visibility of the inner workings and external influences on an AI system. In healthcare, this might mean providing insights into how an AI tool for diagnosing diseases was trained, including the data sources, the developers involved, and the ethical considerations taken into account.

Transparency and explainability are related but distinct concepts in the context of AI, especially in critical fields like healthcare. Transparency is about making the AI system's processes and operations open and accessible, while explainability is about making the outputs of these systems understandable to humans. Both are critical for responsible AI deployment, particularly in sensitive areas like medicine, where trust, ethical considerations, and accurate interpretation are crucial.

Transparency is critical in AI in medicine for several reasons:

- Building Trust and Confidence: Transparent AI systems foster trust and confidence in AI-driven decisions by providing insights into the reasoning behind AI recommendations. This transparency helps alleviate concerns about bias, discrimination, or unintended consequences.
- Enhancing Decision-Making: Transparent AI systems empower healthcare providers to make more informed and personalized decisions by providing a deeper understanding of the factors influencing AI recommendations.
- Promoting Patient Engagement: Transparent AI systems facilitate patient engagement by enabling patients to understand the rationale behind treatment recommendations and participate actively in their care decisions.

- Patient Autonomy: In medicine, patients have the right to understand the reasoning behind their diagnoses and treatments. Transparent AI can help uphold this right by providing clear and understandable explanations for its decisions.
- Regulatory Compliance: In many jurisdictions, medical devices and technologies must be able to explain their decisions to be approved for use. Ensuring that AI technologies are transparent is crucial for regulatory compliance.
- Ensuring Societal Accountability: Transparent AI systems promote societal accountability by enabling public scrutiny and evaluation of AI's role in healthcare. This transparency helps address ethical concerns and ensures responsible AI development.

Despite its importance, achieving transparency in AI in medicine is not without challenges. These include the complexity of AI models, the technical language often used in explanations, and the difficulty of providing explanations that are both accurate and understandable.

To address these challenges, several strategies can be employed:

- Simplification of Models: While complex AI models can provide more accurate predictions, simpler models are often more transparent. Balancing accuracy and transparency is a key challenge in AI in medicine.
- Accessible Documentation: AI systems should be accompanied by clear and accessible documentation that explains their algorithms, data sources, and decision-making processes. This documentation should be tailored to different audiences, including healthcare professionals, patients, and the public.
- Traceability and Auditability: AI systems should be designed with traceability and auditability in mind, allowing users to track the data inputs, intermediate steps, and final outputs of the AI decision-making process. This traceability facilitates accountability and understanding.

- Visualizations and Explanations: AI systems should incorporate visualizations and explanations that aid in understanding the rationale behind AI recommendations. This can include charts, graphs, and annotations that provide context and insights into the AI decision-making process.
- Use of Explainability Techniques: Various techniques have been developed to make AI models more explainable, including feature importance, partial dependence plots, and counterfactual explanations.
- Education and Communication: Providing education and training on AI for healthcare providers and patients can help them better understand AI explanations. Similarly, using clear and non-technical language in explanations can make them more accessible.

Transparency serves as a cornerstone of RAI in medicine, ensuring that AI is used in a way that is open, understandable, and accountable. By fostering transparent AI systems, we can harness the transformative power of AI while upholding ethical principles and ensuring that AI serves the best interests of patients and society. Transparency is not an option; it is a fundamental requirement for responsible AI in medicine.

Privacy and security

Privacy in the context of medical AI refers to the right of patients to have their personal and health data kept confidential and used appropriately. In healthcare, sensitive information ranges from medical records to genetic data, all of which are crucial for AI algorithms in diagnostics, treatment planning, and research. The ethical handling of this data is paramount, as privacy breaches can lead to significant consequences for patients, including discrimination, stigma, and loss of trust in the healthcare system.

Security in medical AI entails protecting health data and AI systems from unauthorized access, breaches, and other cyber threats. The integrity of AI systems in medicine is vital, as any compromise could lead to misdiagnosis, inappropriate treatment recommendations, or leakage of sensitive patient information. Ensuring robust security measures are in place is crucial to safeguarding both the AI systems and the data they process.

Privacy and security are critical in AI in medicine for several reasons:

- Protecting Sensitive Patient Information: Privacy-protective and secure AI systems safeguard sensitive patient data, including medical records, diagnoses, and treatment plans. This protection mitigates the risk of unauthorized access, misuse, and disclosure of personal health information.
- Preserving Patient Autonomy: Privacy-protective AI systems respect patient autonomy by ensuring that patients have control over their data and can make informed decisions about its use. This empowers patients to participate actively in their care and protect their privacy rights.
- Patient Trust: Privacy and security can help build trust in AI technologies among patients. If patients know that their data is being handled securely and their privacy is being respected, they are more likely to accept and use AI technologies.
- Maintaining Public Trust: Secure AI systems foster public trust in the use of AI in healthcare by demonstrating a commitment to data protection and cybersecurity. This trust is crucial for the widespread adoption and acceptance of AI in healthcare.
- Regulatory Compliance: In many jurisdictions, medical devices and technologies must comply with data protection and cybersecurity laws. Ensuring that AI technologies respect privacy and are secure is crucial for regulatory compliance.
- Data Integrity: Security measures help ensure the integrity of the data used by AI systems. This is particularly important in medicine, where the accuracy of patient data can directly impact patient safety and treatment outcomes.

Despite their importance, achieving privacy and security in AI in medicine is not without challenges. These include the sensitivity of medical data, the complexity of AI systems, and the evolving nature of cybersecurity threats.

To address these challenges, several strategies can be employed:

- Data Minimization and Anonymization: Collecting only the necessary data and anonymizing it can help protect patient privacy.
- Access Control and De-identification: AI systems should implement robust access control mechanisms to restrict unauthorized access to patient data. De-identification techniques can be used to protect patient identities while still enabling data analysis and research.
- Encryption and Cybersecurity Measures: AI systems should employ encryption and other cybersecurity measures to protect patient data from cyberattacks and data breaches. Regular security audits and vulnerability assessments are essential to maintain a strong security posture.
- Regular Audits and Updates: Conducting regular security audits and updating AI systems can help identify and address potential security vulnerabilities.
- Ethical Frameworks and Governance: Ethical frameworks and governance structures play a critical role in guiding the responsible use of AI in healthcare. These frameworks should emphasize the importance of privacy and security, providing guidelines for developers, healthcare providers, and policymakers. Governance structures, including oversight committees and regulatory bodies, ensure adherence to these ethical principles and legal standards.

Privacy and security are not just regulatory requirements but fundamental ethical obligations in the application of AI in medicine. They form the bedrock of trust between patients and healthcare providers and are essential for the safe and effective use of AI in healthcare. As we navigate the complexities of digital health, prioritizing privacy and security in medical AI will be crucial for harnessing its full potential while safeguarding the rights and well-being of patients. The path forward requires a concerted effort from all stakeholders in healthcare to ensure that as AI transforms medicine, it does so with the utmost respect for the privacy and security of patient data.

As we conclude this exploration of the key principles of Responsible AI in Medicine, it is evident that the ethical integration of AI into healthcare is a multifaceted and dynamic endeavor. Each principle - from fairness, transparency, and explainability to privacy, security, and beyond - plays a vital role in ensuring that AI serves as a beneficial, trustworthy, and ethical tool in the healthcare landscape.

The integration of AI into medicine is not just a technological advancement; it is a profound responsibility. The principles discussed in this chapter are not standalone concepts but are deeply interconnected. Fairness ensures that AI tools are equitable and unbiased; transparency and explainability build trust and understanding; privacy and security protect the most sensitive patient data while fostering a safe digital health environment. Together, these principles form the foundation of a responsible and ethical approach to AI in medicine.

As AI continues to evolve, so too will the challenges and considerations around its use in healthcare. The future of AI in medicine will be shaped by ongoing research, technological advancements, cross-disciplinary collaboration, and continuous ethical reflection. Policymakers, healthcare providers, AI developers, and patients must work together to navigate these challenges, ensuring that AI is implemented in ways that respect and enhance human health and well-being.

In conclusion, the principles of Responsible AI in Medicine are more than guidelines; they are a commitment to uphold the highest standards of care and ethics in the age of AI. By adhering to these principles, the healthcare community can harness the immense potential of AI to revolutionize medical care, research, and patient outcomes. The journey towards fully realizing the promise of AI in healthcare is complex and ongoing, but by maintaining a steadfast focus on these key principles, we can ensure that AI serves as a force for good, enhancing the health and lives of people around the world.

Chapter 3

Organizing for Responsible AI in Healthcare: A 360 Degree Approach

The advent of Artificial Intelligence (AI) has brought about a paradigm shift in healthcare, offering unprecedented opportunities for improving patient care and health outcomes. However, the successful integration of AI into healthcare requires a comprehensive and strategic approach. This chapter introduces the author's 360-degree approach to organizing for AI in healthcare (HAI360), providing a robust framework for navigating this complex landscape, encompassing organizational charter, organization, competencies, and linkages.

At the core of this approach is the Organizational Charter which establishes the foundation for AI implementation in healthcare. This includes defining the purpose of integrating AI in healthcare, formulating a strategic plan to achieve this purpose, and aligning this plan with the broader AI strategy of the organization, ensuring that AI initiatives are in sync with the overall organizational goals and ethical considerations specific to healthcare.

The Organization segment of Dr. Pillay's model focuses on the design and structure necessary for AI implementation, along with the systems and processes that must be adapted or created. This includes a comprehensive look at organizational redesign, the role of leadership in driving AI initiatives, and the modification of existing systems and processes to support AI integration.

Competencies in the AI era go beyond technical skills. This chapter will cover the essential leadership qualities needed to steer AI initiatives towards success, the cultural shifts required within healthcare organizations to embrace AI, and the individual competencies necessary at various levels of the organization. Emphasis will be placed on ethical decision-making, continuous learning, and adaptability in the face of rapidly evolving AI technologies.

Linkages focuses on the importance of building and maintaining robust connections with both internal and external stakeholders. This encompasses collaboration across different departments within the healthcare organization, as well as partnerships with external entities, including technology providers, regulatory bodies, and patients. The role of these linkages in ensuring ethical, effective, and sustainable AI solutions in healthcare will be thoroughly examined.

Through this comprehensive exploration of the HAI 360 Approach, readers will gain valuable insights into organizing for AI in healthcare, ensuring that AI adoption is not only technologically sound but also ethically responsible and strategically aligned with the overarching goals of healthcare organizations.

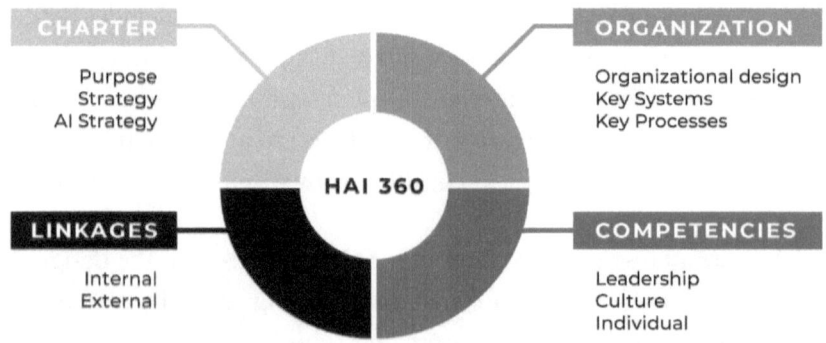

3.1 Organizational Charter

The integration of Artificial Intelligence (AI) in healthcare represents a significant paradigm shift, demanding a strategic and purposeful approach. An Organizational Charter, comprising the organization's purpose, strategic imperatives, and a dedicated AI strategy, is central to this transformation.

The *organizational purpose* defines the fundamental reason for the existence of the healthcare organization. It provides a clear direction for the organization's activities and sets the foundation for its strategic imperatives and AI strategy. For instance, a healthcare organization might define its purpose as "improving patient outcomes through innovative and personalized care."

Strategic imperatives are the critical actions that the organization must take to fulfill its purpose. In the context of AI in healthcare, these could include investing in AI research and development, building partnerships with AI technology providers, or training healthcare providers in the use of AI technologies. For example, a healthcare organization aiming to improve patient outcomes might identify "implementing AI-powered diagnostic tools" as a strategic imperative.

The *AI strategy* outlines the organization's approach to integrating AI in its operations. It includes the organization's goals for AI, the AI technologies it plans to use, and the measures it will take to ensure the responsible use of AI. This strategy should encompass aspects like technology adoption, talent acquisition, infrastructure development, and continuous learning. For instance, the healthcare organization mentioned earlier might outline an AI strategy that involves:

1. Technology Adoption: Partnering with a leading AI healthcare solutions provider to implement the diagnostic tool.
2. Talent Acquisition: Hiring AI specialists and training existing staff to work with AI technologies.

3. Infrastructure Development: Upgrading data storage and processing capabilities to handle large datasets.
4. Continuous Learning: Establishing feedback loops to continually improve the AI tool based on user input and performance data.

Case Study: Mayo Clinic

A real-world example of a healthcare organization that has effectively defined its organizational charter in the context of AI is the Mayo Clinic. The Mayo Clinic's purpose is to provide "the best care to every patient every day through integrated clinical practice, education, and research."

In line with this purpose, the Mayo Clinic has identified several strategic imperatives related to AI. These include advancing the science of healthcare delivery, improving the patient experience, and enhancing the quality and safety of care.

To achieve these strategic imperatives, the Mayo Clinic has developed a comprehensive AI strategy. This strategy includes partnering with AI technology companies, investing in AI research and development, and implementing AI technologies in clinical practice. The Mayo Clinic also places a strong emphasis on the responsible use of AI, with measures in place to ensure the privacy, security, and fairness of its AI initiatives.

Case Study: AI-Powered Diagnostic Assistance at NYU Langone Health

NYU Langone Health, a leading academic medical center, has established a comprehensive AI strategy to enhance its diagnostic capabilities. The organization's AI charter clearly articulates the purpose of AI: to improve diagnostic accuracy and reduce diagnostic errors. This purpose aligns with NYU Langone's overall mission of providing high-quality, patient-centered care.

As part of its AI strategy, NYU Langone has implemented AI-powered diagnostic tools for a variety of medical conditions, including lung

cancer, breast cancer, and stroke. These AI tools assist radiologists in analyzing medical images, providing real-time feedback and highlighting potential abnormalities. By incorporating AI into the diagnostic process, NYU Langone aims to improve diagnostic accuracy, reduce the time to diagnosis, and ultimately improve patient outcomes.

The Organizational Charter in the context of AI in healthcare serves as a fundamental framework guiding organizations in the responsible and effective implementation of AI technologies. As illustrated by the above cases, a well-defined purpose, clear strategic imperatives, and a robust AI strategy are essential for harnessing the potential of AI to revolutionize healthcare. This approach not only ensures alignment with the organization's core values and objectives but also positions it to adapt and thrive in the rapidly evolving landscape of healthcare technology.

3.2 Organization: Designing Structure, Systems, and Processes

The transformative potential of artificial intelligence (AI) in healthcare is undeniable, offering unprecedented opportunities to enhance diagnostics, personalize treatment plans, and improve patient outcomes. Incorporating Artificial Intelligence (AI) into healthcare is not just about technological innovation but also about rethinking the organizational structure, systems, and processes to support this evolution. Responsible AI – AI that is ethical, transparent, and fair – requires an organizational architecture that supports these values. They provide the framework within which AI initiatives are developed, managed, and monitored, ensuring alignment with ethical standards and regulatory requirements.

The organizational structure for responsible AI defines the hierarchy and reporting lines related to AI initiatives. This could include:

Centralized Structure: In a centralized structure, all AI initiatives are managed by a central team or department. This allows for consistent oversight and control over the ethical use of AI.

Mayo Clinic has created a central AI governance body, the AI Oversight Committee, responsible for overseeing the organization's AI initiatives. This committee comprises representatives from various disciplines, including clinical medicine, informatics, ethics, and law. The committee's responsibilities include:

- *Setting AI priorities and strategies: Aligning AI initiatives with the organization's overall mission and strategic goals.*
- *Reviewing AI proposals: Evaluating AI projects for their potential impact, ethical considerations, and feasibility.*
- *Ensuring responsible AI implementation: Overseeing the development, deployment, and monitoring of AI systems to ensure adherence to ethical principles and regulatory requirements.*

Decentralized Structure: In a decentralized structure, individual departments or teams manage their own AI initiatives, with guidance and support from a central AI Ethics Committee or Data Protection Officer.

A good example of a decentralized structure in healthcare is the approach taken by the University of California, San Francisco (UCSF). At UCSF, individual departments such as Radiology, Pathology, and Oncology have their own dedicated teams working on AI initiatives specific to their field. These teams develop and deploy AI models tailored to their department's needs, such as AI algorithms for image analysis in Radiology or predictive models for patient outcomes in Oncology.

While the AI initiatives are managed at the department level, there is also a central AI Ethics Committee that provides guidance and oversight across all departments. This committee is responsible for ensuring that all AI initiatives adhere to ethical guidelines and regulatory standards.

It provides support and resources to the departmental AI teams, helping them navigate ethical considerations and implement best practices in AI.

Additionally, UCSF has a Data Protection Officer who oversees data privacy and security across all AI initiatives. This officer ensures that patient data is handled securely and in compliance with data protection laws, providing an additional layer of oversight and support for the departmental AI teams.

This decentralized structure allows for flexibility and innovation at the department level, while also ensuring ethical and responsible use of AI across the organization. It leverages the specialized expertise of individual departments, while also maintaining a unified approach to AI ethics and data protection.

Hybrid Structure: A hybrid structure combines elements of both centralized and decentralized structures, allowing for flexibility and adaptability in managing AI initiatives.

A good example of a hybrid structure in healthcare is the approach taken by Stanford Health Care. Stanford Health Care has a centralized AI team known as the Clinical Excellence Research Center (CERC), which develops and deploys AI initiatives that are applicable across the entire organization. This team works on projects that have broad applications, such as AI algorithms for predicting patient readmissions or optimizing resource allocation.

In addition to the centralized team, individual departments within Stanford Health Care, such as Radiology or Oncology, have their own dedicated teams working on AI initiatives specific to their field. These teams have the flexibility to develop and deploy AI models tailored to their department's needs, while also benefiting from the resources and oversight provided by the centralized AI team.

This hybrid structure allows for both organization-wide coordination and department-level innovation. The centralized team ensures consistency and alignment with overall organizational goals, while the departmental teams allow for specialization and adaptability to specific contexts. This approach leverages the strengths of both centralized and decentralized structures, providing a flexible and effective framework for managing AI initiatives in healthcare.

Organizational design for responsible AI involves creating roles, teams, and departments that are dedicated to overseeing the ethical use of AI. Cross-functional teams, including AI experts, data scientists, legal advisors, and user experience designers, are crucial in building AI solutions that are not only technically sound but also ethically and socially responsible. This could include:

AI Ethics Committee: An AI Ethics Committee can be established to review and approve AI initiatives, ensuring they comply with ethical guidelines and regulatory requirements. IBM has established an AI Ethics Board, an independent body responsible for advising the company on ethical considerations related to AI development and deployment. The board comprises experts from diverse fields, including technology, law, ethics, and social sciences. Its role includes reviewing AI projects, assessing potential ethical risks, and providing recommendations to ensure that IBM's AI endeavors align with ethical principles.

Data Protection Officer: A Data Protection Officer can be appointed to oversee data privacy and security, ensuring the responsible handling of data used in AI initiatives.

AI Training Team: An AI Training Team can be created to provide education and training on responsible AI to employees, helping them understand the ethical implications of AI and how to use AI responsibly.

Red Teams: Red Teams play a crucial role in the responsible use of AI. A Red Team is an independent group that challenges an organization to improve its effectiveness by assuming an adversarial role. In the context of AI, a Red Team can help identify potential ethical, privacy, or security issues in AI initiatives, providing a critical check on the organization's AI practices. Google AI has established a Red Team, a group of researchers dedicated to identifying and addressing potential biases and vulnerabilities in AI systems. The Red Team works independently of AI development teams, conducting rigorous testing and analysis to uncover potential issues before AI systems are deployed. This approach helps to ensure that AI systems are fair, unbiased, and do not perpetuate harmful stereotypes.

Cases Illustrating Responsible AI Design

IBM's AI Ethics Board: IBM has established an AI Ethics Board that governs its AI initiatives, ensuring they align with ethical principles and societal values.

Google's AI Principles: After facing backlash over its AI projects, Google formulated AI Principles and set up governance structures to ensure responsible development and use of AI.

Microsoft's Responsible AI Standard: Microsoft developed a comprehensive framework, including guidelines, tools, and governance processes, to operationalize responsible AI across its services.

Illustrative Example: AI in Patient Diagnosis

HealthBridge decides to implement an AI system to assist in diagnosing complex diseases. The AI Governance Committee first reviews the project for ethical and practical feasibility. Once approved, a cross-functional team develops the system, guided by the AI Ethics Framework. A Red Team then tests the system, uncovering a tendency to overlook certain symptoms in minority patient groups. The system is refined until it performs accurately across diverse patient demographics. After deployment, the system's performance is continuously monitored, with healthcare professionals providing feedback for further improvements.

Organizational design and structure for responsible AI are about much more than just technical expertise. It requires a holistic approach that includes ethical governance, transparency, diverse and cross-functional teams, and the strategic use of Red Teams to challenge assumptions and identify potential biases. By embedding these elements into the organizational fabric, companies can ensure that their AI initiatives are not only innovative and efficient but also ethically sound and socially responsible.

Key Systems for Responsible AI in Healthcare

Artificial intelligence (AI) has the potential to revolutionize healthcare, offering unprecedented opportunities to enhance diagnostics, personalize treatment plans, and improve patient outcomes. However, the successful integration of AI into healthcare requires a comprehensive and responsible approach. Organizations must implement robust systems to ensure that AI is used ethically, transparently, and responsibly. Artificial intelligence (AI) has the potential to revolutionize healthcare, offering unprecedented opportunities to enhance diagnostics, personalize treatment plans, and improve patient outcomes. However, the successful integration of AI into healthcare requires a comprehensive and responsible approach. Organizations must implement robust systems to ensure that AI is used ethically, transparently, and responsibly

1. Data Governance and Management Systems

AI systems rely heavily on high-quality data for training and decision-making. Healthcare organizations must establish robust data governance and management systems to ensure the quality, integrity, and accessibility of data used for AI. This includes:

- Data Quality Control Measures: Implementing processes to ensure the accuracy, completeness, and consistency of data.
- Data Access and Security Protocols: Establishing mechanisms for controlled access to data while protecting patient privacy and security.

- Data De-identification Practices: Developing techniques for removing patient-identifiable information from data used for AI research and development.
- Ethical Data Usage Framework: This involves establishing clear guidelines on the ethical use of data, including consent protocols, anonymization practices, and fairness in data representation.

Stanford Medicine has implemented a comprehensive data governance framework that encompasses data quality standards, access controls, and de-identification practices. The framework ensures that data used for AI research and development meets ethical standards and protects patient privacy.

Mayo Clinic has implemented a robust data governance framework to ensure the quality, integrity, and accessibility of data used for AI. This framework includes:

- *Data quality control measures: Processes for ensuring the accuracy, completeness, and consistency of data.*
- *Data access and security protocols: Mechanisms for controlled access to data while protecting patient privacy.*
- *Data de-identification practices: Techniques for removing patient-identifiable information from data used for AI research and development.*

The partnership between IBM Watson Health and Mayo Clinic emphasizes ethical data usage, ensuring that patient data used to train AI systems is handled with utmost confidentiality and consent.

2. Cybersecurity Systems

With the increasing use of AI and digital technologies in healthcare, cybersecurity has become a critical concern. Healthcare organizations need to implement robust cybersecurity systems to protect patient data and AI technologies from cyber threats. Cleveland Clinic, for instance, has a dedicated cybersecurity team that works to protect its digital assets, including its AI technologies.

3. AI Model Development and Validation Systems

Healthcare organizations must establish rigorous systems for developing and validating AI models. This includes:

- Model Development Guidelines: Implementing guidelines for selecting appropriate AI algorithms, training models on high-quality data, and evaluating model performance.
- Model Validation and Testing: Conducting rigorous testing and validation of AI models to ensure accuracy, robustness, and fairness.
- Bias Mitigation Strategies: Implementing techniques to identify and mitigate potential biases in AI models.

Mount Sinai has established an AI Validation Center to independently review and validate AI models before they are deployed into clinical practice. The center assesses models for accuracy, robustness, and fairness, ensuring that AI recommendations are reliable and unbiased.

4. AI Deployment and Monitoring Systems

Healthcare organizations must carefully plan and monitor the deployment of AI systems. This includes:

- Integration with Existing Workflows: Integrating AI systems seamlessly into existing clinical workflows to avoid disruptions and ensure efficient operation.
- Continuous Monitoring and Evaluation: Continuously monitoring the performance of AI systems in real-world settings, identifying potential issues, and making adjustments as needed.
- Feedback Mechanisms: Establishing mechanisms for clinicians and patients to provide feedback on AI recommendations, enabling continuous improvement of AI systems.

Kaiser Permanente has developed a comprehensive AI deployment protocol that outlines the steps for integrating AI systems into clinical practice. The protocol includes rigorous testing, clinician training, and ongoing monitoring to ensure the safe and effective use of AI.

5. Transparency and Explainability Systems

Healthcare organizations must strive for transparency in AI development and decision-making. This includes:

- Accessible Documentation: Providing clear and accessible documentation of AI algorithms, decision-making processes, and potential limitations.
- Explainable AI Tools: Integrating explainable AI tools into AI systems to provide visualizations and explanations of AI recommendations.
- Open Communication with Stakeholders: Maintaining open communication with clinicians, patients, and the public about AI initiatives and potential risks and benefits.

Intermountain Healthcare has developed an explainable AI platform that provides clinicians with insights into the rationale behind AI recommendations. The platform helps clinicians understand the factors influencing AI decisions and make informed decisions about patient care.

Mayo Clinic emphasizes transparency and explainability in its AI development and deployment. The organization provides clear documentation of AI algorithms and decision-making processes, allowing clinicians and patients to understand the rationale behind AI recommendations. This transparency fosters trust and enables stakeholders to engage in informed discussions about AI's role in healthcare.

Key Processes for Responsible AI in healthcare

Emerging as a transformative force, artificial intelligence (AI) has permeated various industries, revolutionizing healthcare by enhancing diagnostic accuracy, personalizing treatment plans, and improving patient outcomes. However, alongside its transformative potential lie critical ethical considerations that must be addressed to ensure AI's responsible and beneficial integration into healthcare. Organizations must implement key processes to foster responsible AI practices, ensuring that AI is used ethically, transparently, and responsibly.

AI Model Development Validation Process

Healthcare organizations must establish a rigorous AI lifecycle process that encompasses model development, validation, deployment, and monitoring:

AI Model Development

1. Define the problem or challenge that AI can address.
2. Gather and prepare high-quality data for AI training.
3. Select and implement appropriate AI algorithms.
4. Train AI models on the prepared data.
5. Evaluate model performance using metrics such as accuracy, precision, recall, and F1 score.

AI Model Validation

1. Conduct rigorous testing and validation of AI models to ensure accuracy, robustness, and fairness.
2. Use independent testing sets to avoid overfitting.
3. Assess model performance in real-world scenarios.
4. Identify and address potential biases in AI models.

AI Model Deployment

1. Integrate AI models seamlessly into existing workflows.
2. Provide clear documentation and training for clinicians and other users.
3. Establish continuous monitoring and evaluation of AI models in production.
4. Develop feedback mechanisms to gather input from clinicians and patients.

AI Model Monitoring

1. Continuously monitor the performance of AI models in real-world settings.
2. Identify potential issues and make adjustments as needed.
3. Track the impact of AI models on patient outcomes.
4. Adapt AI models to changing data and clinical practices.
5. Regularly conduct ethical audits of AI systems to assess compliance with established guidelines. This should be coupled with transparent reporting mechanisms for both internal and external stakeholders.
6. Establish channels for employees, users, and other stakeholders to provide feedback on AI systems, ensuring that ethical considerations are continuously updated and refined.

AI in healthcare heavily relies on data. The development process must begin with a **robust data management framework** ensuring data integrity, security, and privacy. This includes implementing standardized procedures for data collection, storage, processing, and sharing. Ensuring data quality and representativeness is critical to develop AI systems that are accurate and unbiased, especially in a field as sensitive as healthcare.

Ethical considerations are paramount in healthcare AI. This involves incorporating principles of fairness, transparency, and accountability into the AI development process. Healthcare organizations must establish ethical guidelines and review boards to oversee AI projects, ensuring that they comply with ethical standards and do not exacerbate existing healthcare disparities.

In healthcare, the focus should be on **augmented intelligence** – AI that supports and enhances human decision-making, rather than replacing it. This approach is particularly suitable for healthcare, where the expertise and judgement of healthcare professionals are irreplaceable. Augmented intelligence can assist in areas like diagnostics, treatment planning, and patient monitoring, enhancing the efficiency and effectiveness of healthcare delivery.

Developing AI in healthcare should be a **collaborative effort** involving not just technologists and data scientists, but also healthcare professionals, patients, ethicists, and policymakers. This multidisciplinary approach ensures that AI systems are designed with a deep understanding of clinical workflows, patient needs, and practical healthcare challenges.

AI systems in healthcare should be designed for **continuous learning and adaptation**. This involves regularly updating the AI algorithms based on new data, feedback from healthcare professionals, and changing healthcare practices. This iterative process ensures that AI systems remain relevant, accurate, and effective over time.

Compliance with healthcare **regulations and safety standards** is crucial. The AI development process must adhere to regulatory requirements such as the Health Insurance Portability and Accountability Act (HIPAA) in the United States and the General Data Protection Regulation (GDPR) in the European Union. Additionally, AI systems must be rigorously tested for safety and efficacy before deployment in clinical settings.

Implementing an AI development process in healthcare is a complex but essential endeavor. It requires a balanced approach that considers technical feasibility, ethical implications, regulatory compliance, and the real-world needs of healthcare professionals and patients. By focusing on these key areas, healthcare organizations can leverage the transformative potential of AI to improve patient care, enhance efficiency, and drive innovation in healthcare.

The Integration of Responsible AI into Clinical and Operational Workflow

However, the successful integration of AI into clinical and operational workflows requires careful consideration of ethical principles, transparency, and patient-centeredness. To harness the power of AI responsibly, healthcare organizations must adopt a structured approach that ensures seamless integration while upholding ethical standards. Before integrating AI into healthcare workflows, it is crucial to assess the specific needs and challenges within a healthcare setting. This involves identifying areas where AI can significantly impact, such as diagnostic accuracy, patient flow management, or administrative efficiency. The suitability of AI solutions for these identified areas must be evaluated to ensure they align with the healthcare facility's goals and capabilities.

1. Understanding the Impact of AI on Clinical Workflows

Clinicians are at the heart of healthcare delivery, and their workflows are often complex and multifaceted. Introducing AI into these workflows must be done thoughtfully to avoid disruptions and ensure that AI complements rather than replaces clinical expertise. Healthcare organizations should:

- Identify opportunities for AI integration: Assess current clinical workflows to identify areas where AI can enhance decision-making, streamline processes, or improve patient outcomes.
- Collaborate with clinicians: Engage clinicians throughout the AI integration process, seeking their input on potential use cases, design considerations, and potential challenges.
- Provide comprehensive training: Equip clinicians with the necessary knowledge and skills to understand, interpret, and interact with AI systems effectively.

2. Addressing Ethical Considerations and Transparency

AI implementation raises critical ethical concerns regarding data privacy, bias mitigation, and algorithmic accountability. Healthcare organizations must prioritize responsible AI practices to foster trust and ensure that AI is used ethically and transparently. This includes:

- Establishing clear ethical guidelines: Develop and implement clear ethical guidelines that govern AI development, deployment, and use.
- Addressing data privacy and security: Implement robust data governance frameworks to protect patient privacy and ensure data security.
- Mitigating biases in AI algorithms: Employ rigorous bias mitigation techniques to identify and address potential biases in AI models.
- Promoting transparency and explainability: Provide clear explanations of AI algorithms and decision-making processes to clinicians and patients.

3. Pilot Implementation and Feedback Loops

Implementing AI solutions should initially be in a pilot phase, allowing for real-time evaluation and adjustments. This phase enables healthcare providers to provide feedback, ensuring that the AI tools effectively support clinical decision-making and operational processes. Continuous feedback loops are essential to refine AI tools and workflows based on practical experiences.

4. Enabling Seamless Integration into Operational Processes

AI integration should not create silos or disrupt existing operational processes. Healthcare organizations should strive for seamless integration that enhances efficiency and collaboration. This includes:

- Assessing operational readiness: Evaluate the organization's readiness for AI integration, including data infrastructure, IT capabilities, and workforce competencies.
- Designing for integration: Ensure that AI systems are designed to integrate seamlessly with existing operational processes and electronic health records (EHRs).
- Training and support for operational staff: Provide training and support to operational staff to ensure they can effectively utilize AI systems in their daily work.

5. Patient-Centeredness and Continuous Monitoring

Throughout the AI integration process, patient-centeredness should remain paramount. Healthcare organizations must ensure that AI systems are used in a way that respects patient autonomy, privacy, and well-being. This includes:

- Obtaining patient consent: Obtain informed consent from patients before using AI to inform their care.
- Maintaining patient control: Ensure that patients retain control over their healthcare decisions and have the ability to opt out of AI-based recommendations.
- Continuous monitoring and evaluation: Continuously monitor the impact of AI on patient outcomes, identify potential unintended consequences, and make adjustments as needed.

Integrating AI into healthcare workflows must adhere to strict ethical guidelines and regulatory compliance. This includes ensuring patient privacy, securing informed consent, and maintaining data security. AI solutions should be transparent, with clear explanations of how they make decisions, to build trust among healthcare professionals and patients.

The integration of responsible AI into clinical and operational workflows has the potential to transform healthcare delivery, improving patient care, enhancing efficiency, and advancing medical knowledge. By adopting a structured approach that prioritizes ethical considerations, transparency, and patient-centeredness, healthcare organizations can harness the power of AI responsibly and ethically, ensuring that AI serves as a valuable tool for improving patient outcomes and advancing the healthcare industry.

The Process for the Procurement of Responsible AI Solutions in Healthcare

The procurement of responsible Artificial Intelligence (AI) solutions in healthcare is a critical process that requires careful consideration and strategic planning. This involves not only assessing the technological capabilities of AI solutions but also ensuring they align with ethical standards, regulatory compliance, and the overall goals of healthcare delivery.

The key steps and considerations in the procurement process of responsible AI solutions in healthcare include:

1. Needs Assessment and Strategic Alignment

- Identify specific AI use cases that align with the organization's overall strategic goals and healthcare mission.
- Assess the organization's readiness for AI implementation, including data maturity, workforce competencies, and cultural factors.
- Establish clear success metrics for AI initiatives to evaluate their impact on patient outcomes and organizational objectives.

2. Vendor Selection and Evaluation

- Conduct thorough research on potential AI vendors, considering their expertise, experience in healthcare, and commitment to responsible AI practices.

- Evaluate vendors' AI solutions based on their performance, scalability, integration capabilities, and adherence to ethical principles.
- Engage in transparent and open communication with vendors to understand their approach to data privacy, security, and bias mitigation.

3. Requirements Definition and Contract Negotiation

- Define detailed requirements for the AI solution, including functional specifications, technical specifications, and ethical considerations.
- Negotiate a contract that clearly outlines the vendor's responsibilities, performance guarantees, and liability for potential risks.
- Establish ongoing communication channels with the vendor to ensure alignment throughout the implementation and post-implementation phases.

4. Implementation and Deployment

- Develop a comprehensive implementation plan that includes data preparation, workflow integration, user training, and change management strategies.
- Establish a rigorous pilot testing and validation process to ensure the AI solution meets performance expectations and adheres to ethical principles.
- Continuously monitor the performance of the AI solution and gather feedback from users to identify areas for improvement.

5. Ongoing Monitoring and Evaluation

- Establish a continuous monitoring framework to track the impact of the AI solution on patient outcomes, organizational efficiency, and ethical considerations.

- Regularly review and evaluate the AI solution to ensure it remains aligned with the organization's needs and advancements in AI technology.
- Maintain open communication with stakeholders, including clinicians, patients, and regulators, to address concerns and ensure transparency.

Procuring responsible AI solutions in healthcare is a multifaceted process that goes beyond technical capabilities. It requires a thorough assessment of vendors, consideration of ethical and regulatory standards, pilot testing, effective training and change management, and continuous post-implementation monitoring. By adhering to these steps, healthcare organizations can successfully integrate AI solutions that not only advance technological capabilities but also uphold the highest standards of patient care and ethical responsibility.

3.3 Competencies Required for the Responsible Deployment of AI in Healthcare

As AI systems become increasingly integral to healthcare delivery, the need for specific competencies at various levels within the organization to ensure responsible deployment is paramount.

Leadership for Responsible AI

AI and machine learning have the power to transform human lives and work for the better, but they can also amplify our worst prejudices and biases. For example, in recent years, multiple cases of biased AI algorithms have unfairly targeted minority groups for crimes they did not commit or facial recognition systems that have difficulty accurately identifying people of color. Such incidents can be harmful to individuals and society as well as to a firm's reputation. Today's consumers will hesitate to buy from a company that doesn't seem in control of its technology or that doesn't protect values like fairness and decency. It falls to the CEO to answer to stakeholders for these incidents and their effects on the firm's brand and financials. Therefore, it is crucial for business leaders to approach AI ethically to avoid such ethical pitfalls, recognize inherent biases and minimize harm. AI is only as good as we lead it so adopting a mindful leadership approach to the way they're designing systems and developing AI technology will result in better outcomes.

These individuals play a pivotal role in steering the ethical and effective integration of AI into healthcare, ensuring that AI is harnessed responsibly to improve patient care and advance medical knowledge. Effective AI leaders in healthcare possess a unique blend of technical expertise, ethical awareness, and leadership acumen that enables them to navigate the complex landscape of AI implementation. The cross-disciplinary nature of RAI demands executive leadership. The CEO can stress to the entire workforce that AI deployed without sufficient governance is a material risk, no matter where it is used in the organization. The democratization of AI by generative AI increases the importance of CEO messaging to instill RAI into corporate culture. RAI becomes integral to strategy when employees do not see the approach as an obstacle to the normal functioning of the business. The CEO has the visibility and authority to convey the message that RAI will enhance business processes and value.

Vision and Strategic Thinking

AI leaders in healthcare must possess a visionary mindset. They need to foresee how AI can transform healthcare and understand the broader implications of AI technologies. This vision is not limited to technological advancement alone but extends to improving patient outcomes, enhancing the efficiency of healthcare services, and addressing systemic healthcare challenges. Visionary leaders are adept at identifying potential AI applications that align with the organization's goals and ethical standards.

Ethical Decision-Making

Given the sensitive nature of healthcare, ethical decision-making is a critical attribute for AI leaders. They must navigate the ethical complexities associated with AI, such as data privacy, bias in algorithms, and the implications of AI decisions on patient care. Responsible AI leaders are committed to upholding ethical standards, ensuring that AI solutions are developed and implemented with a focus on fairness, transparency, and accountability.

AI Technical Knowledge

While AI leaders do not need to be AI experts, they should have a basic understanding of AI technologies and their applications in healthcare. This includes understanding the capabilities and limitations of AI, the data requirements for AI, and the ethical and regulatory considerations related to AI. They should be able to grasp the technical nuances of AI models, assess their potential benefits and limitations, and translate complex technical concepts into comprehensible terms for healthcare professionals and stakeholders. Leaders with interdisciplinary knowledge can effectively bridge the gap between technical teams and healthcare professionals, ensuring that AI solutions are relevant, practical, and aligned with clinical needs.

Change Management Expertise

Implementing AI in healthcare often requires significant changes in workflows, processes, and sometimes organizational culture. AI leaders must have strong change management skills to guide their organizations through these transitions. They should be capable of managing resistance, communicating the benefits of AI effectively, and fostering an environment that embraces technological change while prioritizing patient care.

Collaboration and Communication

AI leaders should have strong collaboration and communication skills. They should be able to collaborate effectively with various stakeholders, including clinicians, data scientists, IT professionals, and administrators. An inclusive approach ensures that diverse perspectives are considered in

AI initiatives, leading to more comprehensive and responsible AI solutions. Collaboration also fosters a culture of shared responsibility and trust, which is crucial for the successful integration of AI in healthcare. They should also be able to communicate the value and benefits of AI in a clear and compelling manner.

Continuous Learning and Adaptability

The field of AI is rapidly evolving, requiring leaders to be committed to continuous learning and adaptation. AI leaders should stay abreast of the latest developments in AI technologies and healthcare trends. This commitment to learning enables them to make informed decisions and keep their organizations at the forefront of innovation in healthcare and responsible AI implementation.

There is an immediate need for action in the healthcare sector regarding Responsible AI (RAI). Some healthcare executives may be inclined to delay RAI implementation until a significant issue arises with an AI system. However, establishing a mature RAI program typically takes about three years. With the increasing deployment of AI in healthcare, now is the critical time for CEOs to commit. Implementing RAI before scaling AI operations can optimize technology investments and enhance patient care. In our experience, healthcare organizations that prioritize RAI before expanding their AI capabilities encounter fewer system failures and extract greater value from AI technologies.

For a successful RAI program, several steps are essential, and the responsibility ultimately lies with the CEO. A leader's direct involvement ensures that AI usage aligns with RAI principles, integrating them into the core of the healthcare organization's culture and operations.

Firstly, a coherent *strategy must align RAI with the healthcare organization's values.* The CEO should articulate how ethical AI usage, adherence to corporate codes of conduct, and AI applications are in harmony with the organization's mission and values. This involves more than just stating principles; it requires a detailed plan to integrate RAI into governance, processes, tools, and the organizational culture.

Secondly, appoint a senior *leader responsible for RAI execution*. The CEO's endorsement of RAI is pivotal, but it's equally crucial to assign a dedicated leader to implement the strategy and tackle challenges. This role could be filled by the Chief Risk Officer, the leader of ESG initiatives, or a Chief AI Officer. Alternatively, creating a new role, such as Chief AI Ethics Officer, might be necessary. The CEO should not only appoint but also provide ample resources to this leader and hold them accountable for the success of the RAI program.

Thirdly, *embed RAI within cross-functional risk/governance processes*. When planning AI projects, input from multidisciplinary teams is essential to assess risks and establish safeguards. Many organizations form a special committee for RAI, but it should be integrated into broader risk/governance processes, not isolated. Representatives from the RAI committee should participate in existing forums like the management risk committee or the product approval committee. There should be clear escalation paths in governance processes that lead back to the CEO.

Lastly, the CEO must *actively communicate and prioritize RAI*. This includes highlighting RAI in speeches, emails, board meetings, and explaining its importance to stakeholders, including patients, partners, industry groups, and regulators.

Just as CEOs in healthcare prioritize ESG, DEI, and cybersecurity, RAI should receive equal emphasis. This commitment not only enhances AI deployments but also aligns with broader organizational goals, ensuring responsible innovation and strengthening the healthcare system overall.

In the spirit of the Hippocratic Oath, which has guided physicians for centuries to practice medicine ethically and responsibly, we propose a similar oath for leaders overseeing the deployment and management of Responsible AI(RAI) in healthcare. This oath serves as a moral compass, ensuring that RAI is used to enhance patient care, uphold privacy, and promote well-being, without causing harm.

The AI Stewardship Pledge for Healthcare

First, Do No Harm: I pledge to prioritize patient safety and well-being in all RAI applications, ensuring that these technologies are used to enhance, not compromise, the quality of healthcare.

Respect for Privacy and Confidentiality: I vow to uphold the highest standards of data privacy and confidentiality, ensuring that all RAI systems comply with ethical guidelines and legal regulations in handling patient information.

Commitment to Fairness and Non-Discrimination: I promise to actively work against biases in RAI algorithms and data sets, striving for equitable and fair treatment of all patients, regardless of their background.

Transparency and Accountability: I shall maintain transparency in RAI operations and decision-making processes, ensuring that AI systems are explainable and that I am accountable for their outcomes.

Collaboration and Inclusivity: I pledge to foster a culture of collaboration and inclusivity, engaging with a diverse range of stakeholders, including healthcare professionals, patients, and ethicists, to guide responsible RAI implementation.

Continual Learning and Adaptation: I commit to staying informed about advancements in AI and healthcare, adapting RAI applications to emerging knowledge and technologies while upholding ethical standards.

Promotion of Public Trust: I will endeavor to build and maintain public trust in RAI technologies, ensuring that their use in healthcare is aligned with societal values and expectations.

Advocacy for Patient-Centered Care: I promise to ensure that RAI technologies are used to enhance patient-centered care, supporting the needs and preferences of patients while complementing the expertise of healthcare providers.

Ethical Leadership and Influence: I vow to lead by example, promoting ethical practices in the use of RAI in healthcare, and influencing others in my field to follow these principles.

Responsibility Towards Societal Impact: I acknowledge my responsibility towards the broader societal impact of RAI in healthcare, and I pledge to work towards solutions that benefit the health and well-being of communities.

This oath for leaders in SAI in healthcare serves as a foundational guide to navigate the complex ethical landscape of AI in medicine. By adhering to these principles, leaders can ensure that the integration of SAI in healthcare respects human dignity, promotes health equity, and contributes positively to the advancement of medical care for all.

Cultural Competencies for Responsible AI

Artificial intelligence (AI) has emerged as a transformative force in healthcare, revolutionizing disease diagnosis, treatment personalization, and operational efficiency. However, the successful integration of AI into healthcare requires a comprehensive approach that extends beyond technical expertise and encompasses cultural competencies to ensure ethical, equitable, and responsible AI implementation.

Cultivating Ethical Awareness and Discourse

AI development and deployment raise critical ethical concerns regarding data privacy, bias mitigation, and algorithmic accountability. Fostering a culture of ethical awareness and discourse is paramount to address these concerns. Healthcare organizations should encourage open discussions about ethical dilemmas, potential biases, and the impact of AI on patients, clinicians, and society. This culture should encourage diverse perspectives and collaboration among clinicians, data scientists, ethicists, and patients, enabling informed decision-making and ensuring that AI is used responsibly.

- ➢ Establish ethics committees and working groups: Create dedicated committees or working groups that bring together clinicians, data scientists, ethicists, and legal experts to discuss ethical considerations and develop guidelines for AI implementation.
- ➢ Organize ethics workshops and seminars: Conduct regular workshops and seminars on AI ethics to educate healthcare professionals about ethical principles, potential biases, and responsible AI practices.
- ➢ Encourage open communication and debate: Foster a culture of open communication and encourage lively debates about the ethical implications of AI in healthcare settings.
- ➢ Redefine success metrics to include ethical considerations. This means not just evaluating AI systems based on accuracy or efficiency but also on how well they align with ethical principles.
- ➢ Design incentive structures that reward not only high performance but also adherence to ethical practices. This could include recognition programs, career advancement opportunities, or other benefits.

Prioritizing Transparency and Explainability

Transparency and explainability are essential pillars of responsible AI. Healthcare organizations should strive to make AI systems transparent and understandable, providing clear explanations of how AI algorithms work, the factors influencing AI recommendations, and the limitations of AI models. This transparency fosters trust among clinicians, patients, and the public, enabling informed decision-making and ensuring that AI is used responsibly and effectively.

- ➢ Develop clear documentation and explanations: Provide comprehensive documentation and explanations of AI algorithms, decision-making processes, and limitations.

- Implement explainable AI (XAI) techniques: Utilize XAI techniques to make AI models more transparent and understandable, allowing clinicians and patients to understand the rationale behind AI recommendations.
- Engage in open dialogue with stakeholders: Engage in open dialogue with clinicians, patients, and the public to address concerns and provide clear explanations of AI applications.

Embracing Patient-Centeredness and Inclusivity

AI implementation should always prioritize patient well-being and patient-centeredness. Healthcare organizations should embed patient-centeredness into their AI initiatives, ensuring that AI systems align with patient values, preferences, and autonomy. This involves involving patients in AI development processes, incorporating patient feedback, and ensuring that AI recommendations are consistent with patient-centered care principles. Additionally, organizations should consider cultural sensitivities and ensure that AI systems are inclusive and do not perpetuate societal inequities.

- Involve patients in AI development: Include patients in the AI development process, seeking their feedback on AI applications and ensuring that their needs and preferences are considered.
- Conduct patient-centered impact assessments: Evaluate the impact of AI on patient outcomes, considering factors such as patient satisfaction, clinical effectiveness, and potential disparities.
- Address cultural sensitivities and bias: Train healthcare professionals to identify and address cultural sensitivities and potential biases in AI algorithms and applications.

Encouraging Continuous Learning and Adaptability

The rapid evolution of AI technology necessitates a culture of continuous learning and adaptability. Healthcare organizations should encourage their workforce to stay up-to-date with the latest AI advancements, ethical considerations, and best practices. This can be achieved through training programs, workshops, and a supportive environment that encourages individuals to explore new AI applications and adapt to the changing landscape of AI in healthcare.

- ➢ Establish continuous AI education programs: Develop and implement ongoing AI education programs for clinicians, data scientists, and other healthcare professionals.
- ➢ Promote attendance at AI conferences and workshops: Encourage healthcare professionals to attend AI conferences and workshops to stay up-to-date on the latest advancements and best practices.
- ➢ Create a supportive learning environment: Foster a supportive learning environment that encourages individuals to explore new AI applications and adapt to the changing landscape of AI in healthcare.

Promoting Accountability and Responsibility

Accountability and responsibility are paramount in responsible AI implementation. Healthcare organizations should establish clear accountability structures that delineate responsibilities for AI development, deployment, and monitoring. This includes identifying individuals or teams responsible for addressing potential ethical issues, ensuring data privacy, and mitigating biases in AI models. Small hospitals might not have all the resources needed for implementing ethical AI. Collaborating with industry partners, participating in forums, and learning from case studies can be beneficial.

- ➢ Establish clear accountability structures: Define clear roles and responsibilities for AI development, deployment, monitoring, and governance.
- ➢ Implement robust AI governance frameworks: Develop and implement comprehensive AI governance frameworks that outline ethical principles, risk management procedures, and accountability mechanisms.

> Conduct regular AI audits and assessments: Conduct regular audits and assessments of AI systems to identify potential issues, ensure compliance with ethical guidelines, and evaluate the impact on patient outcomes.

Fostering Open Communication and Collaboration

Open communication and collaboration are crucial for responsible AI implementation. Healthcare organizations should foster a collaborative environment where diverse perspectives and expertise are valued. This involves encouraging open communication among clinicians, data scientists, ethicists, patients, and other stakeholders, enabling collective problem-solving and informed decision-making.

> Create interdisciplinary AI teams: Establish interdisciplinary AI teams that bring together clinicians, data scientists, ethicists, and other experts to collaborate on AI projects.
> Encourage open communication channels: Establish open communication channels and platforms for sharing ideas, concerns, and feedback related to AI implementation.
> Host regular AI forums and meetings: Organize regular AI forums and meetings to facilitate discussions, foster collaboration, and address emerging challenges.
> Engage a diverse range of stakeholders, including users, regulatory bodies, and civil society groups, in the development and deployment of AI systems. This helps to ensure a variety of perspectives and needs are considered.

Cultural competencies are essential for responsible AI implementation in healthcare. By cultivating ethical awareness, prioritizing transparency, embracing patient-centeredness, encouraging continuous learning, promoting accountability, and fostering open communication, healthcare organizations can harness the transformative power of AI while upholding ethical principles, ensuring patient well-being, and advancing the future of healthcare.

Individual level competencies for Responsible AI

In a world increasingly shaped by artificial intelligence (AI), equipping individuals with responsible AI literacy has become imperative. Beyond mere technical understanding, responsible AI literacy encompasses a diverse set of critical competencies that enable individuals to navigate the complexities of AI technology with awareness, ethical judgment, and informed action.

Technical skills

The foundation of responsible AI literacy lies in a grasp of the technical aspects of AI, such as data science, machine learning, natural language processing, computer vision, and robotics. You need to understand how AI systems work, what are their strengths and limitations, and how to optimize their performance and accuracy. You also need to be familiar with the tools and frameworks that enable you to build and test AI applications, such as Python, and AWS. Technical skills are essential for creating AI solutions that are reliable, scalable, and secure.

Ethical skills

The second skill you need is the ability to identify and address the ethical implications of AI, such as fairness, accountability, transparency, privacy, and human dignity. You need to be aware of the potential biases, risks, and harms that AI can cause or amplify, such as discrimination, manipulation, surveillance, and displacement. You also need to be able to apply ethical principles and frameworks, such as the AI Ethics Guidelines of the European Commission or the IEEE Ethically Aligned Design, to guide your decision making and actions. Ethical skills are crucial for ensuring that AI respects human rights and values. By developing this ethical lens, individuals can critically evaluate AI applications and advocate for responsible use.

Social skills

Effectively communicating about AI is crucial for raising awareness, fostering collaboration, and promoting responsible use. Responsible AI literacy empowers individuals to communicate complex AI concepts in clear and understandable language, engage in constructive dialogue with diverse stakeholders, and effectively advocate for ethical and responsible AI development and deployment. You need to be able to listen and empathize with their perspectives, needs, and expectations, as well as to explain and justify your AI solutions in a clear and accessible way. You also need to be able to work in teams and networks, leveraging the collective intelligence and creativity of different disciplines and backgrounds. Social skills are vital for building trust and engagement with AI.

Environmental skills

The fourth skill you need is the awareness and knowledge of the environmental impacts of AI, such as energy consumption, carbon footprint, waste generation, and biodiversity loss. You need to be able to measure and monitor the environmental costs and benefits of your AI solutions, as well as to adopt best practices and standards for reducing and mitigating them. You also need to be able to explore and innovate ways of using AI for environmental protection and restoration, such as climate change mitigation, wildlife conservation, and circular economy. Environmental skills are key for making AI sustainable and regenerative.

Critical Thinking and Problem-Solving Skills

critical thinking and problem-solving skills are essential for navigating the complexities and challenges associated with this technology. Responsible AI literacy fosters these skills by encouraging individuals to analyze information critically, identify potential risks and opportunities, and develop creative solutions to AI-related problems. You need to be able to analyze and evaluate the health and healthcare issues that AI can address or create, using evidence, logic, and reasoning. You need to be able to question and challenge the assumptions, values, and goals that underlie your AI solutions, as well as to recognize and avoid the pitfalls and fallacies that can affect your thinking and judgment. You also need to be able to learn from feedback, experience, and research, and to update and improve your AI solutions accordingly. Critical skills are important for making AI relevant and adaptive.

Creative skills and Human Centered Design

The sixth skill you need is the talent to imagine and generate novel and valuable ideas and solutions for health and healthcare issues using AI. You need to be able to combine and integrate different sources of information, inspiration, and insight, as well as to experiment and prototype different possibilities and alternatives. You also need to be able to express and share your ideas and solutions in compelling and engaging ways, using storytelling, visualization, and other media. Creative skills are essential for making AI innovative and transformative.

Responsible AI prioritizes human values and needs throughout its development and implementation. Cultivating a human-centered design approach is crucial for ensuring that AI systems are beneficial and empowering for individuals. This requires understanding the impact of AI on human behavior, designing AI systems that are inclusive and accessible, and ensuring that AI complements and enhances human capabilities rather than replacing them

Legal and Policy Awareness

This entails regulatory knowledge which is an awareness of the laws and policies governing AI use ensures compliance and ethical application. Additional it requires knowledge of compliance and safety standards of industry-specific regulations and safety standards essential for risk management.

Developing responsible AI literacy is no longer a luxury, but a necessity for navigating the complex and transformative world shaped by AI. By fostering the critical competencies outlined above, individuals can become informed and engaged citizens, contributing to a future where AI is harnessed for good, upholding ethical principles, and empowering individuals and communitie

Chapter 4

AI Governance for Healthcare Leaders

Given the swift progress and widespread implementation of AI systems in healthcare, there is an increasing demand from healthcare organizations, practitioners, and regulatory bodies to establish effective oversight for these technologies. As healthcare systems increasingly integrate AI to enhance patient care, diagnostics, treatment planning, and operational efficiency, instances of AI-related issues continue to surface.

In healthcare, AI systems are encountering challenges such as bias in diagnosis, concerns over patient data ownership and privacy, accuracy in medical predictions, and cybersecurity risks. These challenges pose significant risks, ranging from misdiagnoses to breaches in patient confidentiality, potentially leading to serious consequences for patient safety and trust. The implementation of robust AI Governance is crucial in addressing these issues, enabling healthcare organizations to harness the full benefits of AI while mitigating potential harms.

AI Governance in healthcare, though still a developing field, encompasses a range of measures from regulatory compliance to voluntary best practices within organizations. These governance efforts are becoming essential for the safe, ethical, and responsible use of AI in healthcare settings. Recent analyses suggest that the responsibility for AI Governance should ultimately be assumed by top-level healthcare executives, as it involves critical aspects such as patient trust, ethical use of AI in clinical settings, stakeholder interests, and adherence to healthcare regulations.

As an evolving and complex domain, AI Governance in healthcare is being shaped by healthcare policymakers, legal experts, medical societies, and industry leaders. Recognizing the challenges in initiating AI Governance practices, this paper aims to provide a strategic overview of various governance mechanisms, offering guidance to healthcare leaders in navigating this intricate and rapidly changing landscape.

Navigating AI Governance

When establishing an AI Governance practice, it's important to understand the scope and purpose of each AI Governance instrument. The figure below summarizes the different types of AI governance mechanisms, which are detailed further in the sections that follow.

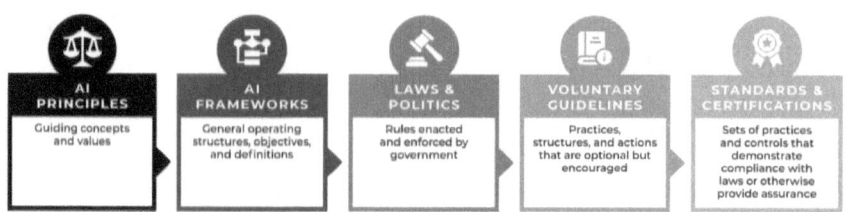

The Spectrum of AI Governance

AI Principles

Given the rapid progression and increasing application of AI in healthcare, there is an urgent need for oversight mechanisms to ensure the responsible deployment of these technologies. Healthcare organizations, practitioners, and regulators are advocating for the establishment of guidelines and frameworks to address potential risks associated with AI in healthcare.

From 2016 to 2019, governments and international entities, like the Organization for Economic Cooperation and Development (OECD), recognized critical issues related to the growing use of AI in healthcare. Acknowledging AI's profound implications on health and wellness, these bodies have engaged in multi-stakeholder processes to develop guiding principles for AI's ethical and effective use in healthcare.

Foundational initiatives such as the OECD's AI Principles, Asilomar Principles, IEEE's Ethically Aligned Design, and the Montréal Declaration have set benchmarks and inspired governance mechanisms, including laws, corporate policies, and standards specific to healthcare. These frameworks often emphasize themes crucial to healthcare, such as patient privacy, fairness and equity in treatment, accuracy of medical AI systems, transparency and explainability, accountability, and the necessity of human oversight in clinical decision-making.

While establishing these principles is a significant first step in discussing effective AI oversight in healthcare, they often represent high-level, aspirational ideals. Healthcare practitioners developing AI-based diagnostic tools, treatment plans, and patient management systems need actionable guidance on implementing these principles and managing potential trade-offs.

Healthcare organizations should develop AI governance programs that either build upon these existing principles or align closely with them. The principles should be tailored to reflect the specific nature of the healthcare industry, the domain of application, and the types of AI systems being deployed. They should also resonate with the organization's mission and values, guiding healthcare providers on what is essential and the types of AI applications to pursue.

The guiding principles and values that should inform the responsible use of AI in healthcare include:

Principle 1: Beneficence and Non-Maleficence

The principle of beneficence requires that AI technologies in healthcare should aim to benefit patients and improve health outcomes. This includes improving the accuracy and speed of diagnoses, enhancing the effectiveness of treatments, and reducing the burden on healthcare professionals.

Conversely, the principle of non-maleficence requires that AI technologies should not harm patients or exacerbate health disparities. This includes avoiding biases in AI algorithms that could lead to unfair treatment or outcomes for certain groups of patients.

Principle 2: Autonomy and Informed Consent

The principle of autonomy requires that patients should have the right to make informed decisions about their healthcare, including the use of AI technologies. This requires clear and understandable explanations of how AI technologies work, what data they use, and what risks they entail.

Informed consent is a key aspect of respecting patient autonomy. Patients should be fully informed about the use of AI in their care and should have the opportunity to opt out if they wish.

Principle 3: Privacy and Confidentiality

The principle of privacy and confidentiality requires that AI technologies should respect the privacy of patients and protect their health data. This includes using secure and anonymized data storage and transmission methods, and ensuring that AI algorithms do not inadvertently reveal sensitive information.

Principle 4: Justice and Equity

The principle of justice and equity requires that AI technologies should be used to promote fairness and equity in healthcare. This includes ensuring that AI technologies are accessible and beneficial to all patients, regardless of their socioeconomic status, race, gender, or geographic location.

Principle 5: Transparency and Accountability

The principle of transparency requires that AI technologies should be transparent in their workings and decision-making processes. This includes providing clear explanations of how AI algorithms make predictions or recommendations.

The principle of accountability requires that there should be mechanisms in place to hold AI developers and users accountable for the outcomes of AI technologies. This includes establishing guidelines and regulations for the development and use of AI in healthcare, and setting up systems for monitoring and auditing AI technologies.

Principle 6: Public Engagement and Trust

Building public trust in AI is crucial for its successful integration into healthcare. Open dialogue and engagement with diverse stakeholders, including patients, healthcare professionals, and policymakers, are essential to address concerns, educate the public about AI's potential benefits, and foster a shared understanding of its ethical implications.

Principle 7: Continuous Learning and Improvement

The dynamic nature of AI necessitates ongoing learning and improvement. Healthcare institutions and developers must continuously update their knowledge, adapt to evolving technologies, and actively seek feedback from patients and clinicians to refine AI applications and ensure their continued relevance and effectiveness.

Review Microsoft principles[5] here: https://www.microsoft.com/en-us/ai/principles-and-approach

---

[5] https://www.microsoft.com/en-us/ai/principles-and-approach

Review Google principles[6] here: https://ai.google/responsibility/responsible-ai-practices/

Review OECD principles[7] here: https://oecd.ai/en/ai-principles

Review Asilomar Principles[8] here: https://futureoflife.org/open-letter/ai-principles/

AI Frameworks

AI governance principles and AI governance frameworks are both crucial components of responsible AI, but they serve different purposes and operate at different levels.

AI Governance Principles are high-level ethical guidelines that outline the values and standards that should guide the development and use of AI technologies. They are often abstract and aspirational, providing a vision of what responsible AI should look like. Examples of AI governance principles include fairness, transparency, accountability, privacy, and beneficence.

On the other hand, an AI Governance Framework is a more detailed and practical tool that translates these high-level principles into actionable policies, procedures, and controls. It provides a structured approach to implementing the principles in the real world, often including mechanisms for monitoring compliance, assessing performance, and addressing violations. A framework might include specific guidelines for data handling, model training, algorithmic transparency, user consent, and more.

In essence, while principles provide the 'what' (the ethical standards we aim to uphold), the framework provides the 'how' (the practical steps to achieving those standards). Both are necessary for the responsible and ethical use of AI. The progression from principles to a framework

---

[6] https://ai.google/responsibility/responsible-ai-practices/
[7] https://oecd.ai/en/ai-principles
[8] https://futureoflife.org/open-letter/ai-principles/

is a step-by-step process that moves from conceptual understanding to practical application:

1. Principle Interpretation: Each principle is meticulously analyzed and interpreted to derive actionable guidance for AI development. For example, the principle of fairness requires identifying potential biases in data and algorithms and implementing mitigation strategies.
2. Policy Development: Based on the interpretation, specific policies are formulated to translate principles into concrete actions. These policies may encompass data governance, user consent mechanisms, transparency reporting requirements, and accountability measures.
3. Implementation Strategies: Practical implementation strategies are devised to operationalize the policies effectively. This may involve training programs for developers, ethical review committees for new AI applications, and accessible user interfaces for explaining AI decisions.
4. Monitoring and Evaluation: Ongoing monitoring and evaluation mechanisms are established to assess the effectiveness of the framework in achieving the desired outcomes. This includes evaluating the impact of AI on individuals, communities, and the environment, identifying areas for improvement, and continuously adapting the framework to evolving technologies and societal needs.
5. Stakeholder Engagement: Open communication and engagement with diverse stakeholders, including developers, policymakers, users, and civil society organizations, are crucial throughout the framework development and implementation process. This ensures inclusivity, diverse perspectives, and collective ownership of responsible AI practices.
6. Continuous Improvement: Recognizing the dynamic nature of AI and society, the framework should be a living document, constantly evolving and adapting to address emerging challenges and opportunities. This necessitates ongoing research, innovation,

and collaborative efforts to continuously improve the responsible development and deployment of AI.

In this way, the high-level principles are translated into actionable steps, forming a comprehensive and practical framework for responsible AI.

The benefits of a framework include:

- Provides a comprehensive and structured approach to guide responsible AI development and deployment.
- Promotes ethical considerations throughout the AI lifecycle, from design to deployment and post-implementation evaluation.
- Ensures accountability and responsibility for the societal impact of AI applications.
- Fosters trust and public confidence in AI through transparency, explainability, and user control.
- Maximizes the positive impact of AI by addressing critical societal challenges and promoting inclusivity and well-being.

Review National Institute of Standards and Technology (NIST) AI Risk Management Framework[9] here: https://www.responsible.ai/post/understanding-the-national-institute-of-standards-and-technology-nist-ai-risk-management-framework

Review OECD Framework for the Classification of AI systems here: https://www.oecd.org/publications/oecd-framework-for-the-classification-of-ai-systems-cb6d9eca-en.htm

---

[9] https://www.responsible.ai/post/understanding-the-national-institute-of-standards-and-technology-nist-ai-risk-management-framework

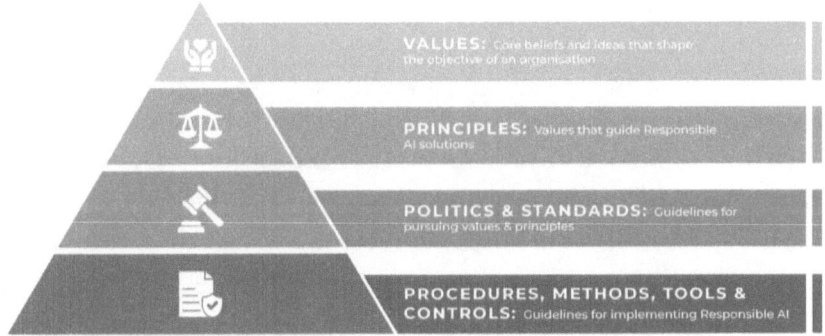

A Framework for Defining Responsible AI Initiatives

Laws and Regulations

The rapid development and deployment of Artificial Intelligence (AI) raise complex questions about responsible development and use. To address these concerns, different approaches coexist and complement each other, each playing a distinct role in shaping the future of AI.

Laws and regulations represent the most formal and authoritative approach. They are enacted by legislative bodies and carry the force of law, imposing mandatory obligations and potential penalties for non-compliance. Laws often focus on specific areas of concern, such as data privacy, algorithmic bias, or autonomous weapons, and provide detailed requirements for developers and users of AI systems. Their legally binding nature ensures a baseline level of compliance and offers a strong foundation for responsible AI development. AI laws and regulations often focus on specific areas deemed most critical, leading to a less comprehensive approach compared to frameworks. As legislative processes are inherently slow and deliberate, adjusting AI laws and regulations to keep pace with rapid technological advancements can be challenging.

Examples of AI Laws and Regulations Include:

USA:

Algorithmic Justice and Anti-Discrimination Act (AJADA): This proposed federal law prohibits discrimination based on protected characteristics in AI algorithms and requires transparency and explainability in their development and use.

California Consumer Privacy Act (CCPA) and Virginia Consumer Data Protection Act (VCDPA): These state laws grant consumers rights to access, correct, and delete their personal data, including data collected by AI systems.

New York City Automated Employment Decision Tools Law: This law requires employers to conduct bias audits of AI-powered hiring tools before using them.

Federal Trade Commission (FTC) Guides Against Deception and Unfairness: These guidelines apply to AI-powered services and products, requiring them to be truthful, not deceptive, and avoid unfair

Note that in the USA, AI is regulated both at federal and state level, so it is imperative that both are studied.

EU:

General Data Protection Regulation (GDPR): This regulation grants individuals control over their personal data and requires companies to be transparent about how they collect and use data, including data used in AI systems.

Artificial Intelligence Act (proposed): This proposed regulation sets out comprehensive rules for the development, deployment, and use of AI systems, including requirements for risk management, human oversight, and transparency.

Member state laws: Several EU member states have enacted their own AI-specific laws, such as Germany's Act on the Transparency of Algorithmic Decision-Making Processes in Administrative Procedures.

These different approaches tom AI Governance are not mutually exclusive but rather complementary. AI laws provide a strong legal foundation, policies offer broader guidance, frameworks provide a structured roadmap, and principles offer a high-level ethical vision. By working together, these different approaches can create a robust and comprehensive framework for ensuring responsible AI development and use.

Here is a table summarizing the key differences between AI laws, policies, frameworks, and principles:

Feature	AI Laws & Regulations	AI Frameworks	AI Principles
Legally binding	Yes	No	No
Scope	Specific	Comprehensive	Broad
Detail	Specific and detailed	Structured set of guidelines	General and aspirational
Flexibility	Least flexible	Flexible and adaptable	Most flexible
Enforceability	Enforceable through legal system	No direct enforcement mechanisms	No direct enforcement mechanisms
Example	GDPR (General Data Protection Regulation)	EU Ethics Guidelines for Trustworthy AI	Asilomar AI Principles

Civil Society and AI Governance

Governments and corporations are critical actors in AI governance, but we need civil society at the center. Civil society organizations' (CSOs) main purpose is to advocate for and protect the public interest by actively engaging with those powers and exercising oversight. Civil society voices can have a powerful role in counterbalancing government and corporations' positions by expanding the dialogue to include broader societal interests, including the rule of law, and factor in developing legal and regulatory frameworks that will shape AI governance. We need diverse voices to scrutinize how foundation models and generative AI intersect with our legal, judicial, and regulatory systems.

Artificial Intelligence (AI) in medicine promises to revolutionize healthcare, offering tools that can enhance diagnostics, streamline patient care, and even predict health outcomes. But with this promise comes profound ethical, societal, and governance challenges. As we stand at the intersection of medicine and technology, one thing becomes increasingly clear: civil society must be at the heart of medical AI governance. Here's why.

- AI in healthcare is not just a technological issue; it's a societal one. It affects everyone - patients, healthcare providers, and the general public. Therefore, decisions about its use and governance should not be left solely to technologists, physicians or policymakers. Civil society, representing the interests of the public, has a vital role to play.
- Medical AI, while technologically advanced, operates in a domain deeply rooted in human values, trust, and ethics. Whether it's diagnosing diseases or recommending treatments, the decisions made by AI have direct human implications. Civil society, representing diverse voices and ethical considerations, can ensure that AI solutions are not just technically sound but morally justifiable. Civil society can advocate for ethical AI use, ensuring that AI applications respect human rights and are used for public good. They can raise awareness about the implications of AI, educating the public about their rights and potential risks.
- The rapidly evolving landscape of medical AI requires agile policy frameworks. Civil society, with its pulse on societal needs and challenges, can influence policy-making, ensuring that regulations are both progressive and protective of patient rights. Civil society organizations can influence policy-making, ensuring that regulations protect public interests. They can provide valuable insights from the ground level, helping to shape policies that are practical and effective.

- As AI models become intricate, there's a growing need for transparency. Civil society can act as a watchdog, ensuring that AI developers and healthcare institutions remain accountable. By demanding clear explanations for AI decisions, they can ensure that the technology remains comprehensible and accountable. Civil society plays a crucial role in holding stakeholders accountable. They can monitor AI applications in healthcare, report unethical practices, and ensure that those responsible are held accountable.
- AI in medicine should be equitable, catering to the needs of all sections of society. Civil society can play a pivotal role in ensuring that AI solutions are inclusive, addressing the needs of marginalized communities and ensuring that biases, often inherent in datasets, don't perpetuate healthcare disparities.
- While technologists and medical experts bring vital domain-specific knowledge, civil society brings a broader perspective. They can bridge the gap between technical jargon and real-world implications, ensuring that the wider public understands the potential risks and benefits of medical AI. Civil society can advocate for ethical AI use, ensuring that AI applications respect human rights and are used for public good. They can raise awareness about the implications of AI, educating the public about their rights and potential risks.

Here are some examples of how CSOs are already working to promote responsible AI in medicine:

- The Algorithmic Justice League is a CSO that works to ensure that algorithms are used in a fair and just way. They have developed a number of resources to help policymakers and the public understand the potential for bias in AI systems.
- The Center for Democracy and Technology is a CSO that works to promote responsible innovation in technology. They have published a number of reports on the ethical implications of AI in healthcare.
- The Partnership on AI is a non-profit organization that brings together companies, universities, and nonprofits to work on the

responsible development and use of AI. They have developed a number of resources to help organizations implement responsible AI practices.

There are a number of ways to incorporate civil society organizations (CSOs) in medical AI governance. Here are a few suggestions:

- Establish CSOs as members of medical AI governance bodies: CSOs should have a seat at the table when it comes to making decisions about how medical AI is developed, deployed, and used. This will help to ensure that the voices of the public are heard and that ethical concerns are taken into account.
- Provide funding for CSOs to work on medical AI governance: CSOs need resources to be able to do the important work of educating the public, advocating for responsible AI policies, monitoring the use of medical AI, and developing and promoting ethical guidelines. Governments and philanthropic organizations can provide funding to support this work.
- Partner with CSOs on medical AI governance initiatives: Governments, policymakers, and other stakeholders can partner with CSOs on specific medical AI governance initiatives. For example, they could work with CSOs to develop ethical guidelines for medical AI or to monitor the use of medical AI for bias.

Here are some specific examples of how CSOs are being incorporated in medical AI governance today:

- In the United Kingdom, the National Health Service (NHS) has established a Centre for AI in Healthcare. The Centre has a CSO advisory group that provides input on the ethical and social implications of AI in healthcare.
- In the United States, the Food and Drug Administration (FDA) has established a Digital Health Center of Excellence. The Center has a CSO engagement program that works with CSOs to get their input

on the development and regulation of digital health technologies, including AI-powered medical tools.
- The European Commission has established a High-Level Expert Group on Artificial Intelligence. The Group includes representatives from CSOs, industry, academia, and government. The Group is tasked with developing recommendations on the responsible development and use of AI in Europe.

The fusion of AI and medicine is not just a technological transformation but a societal one. While AI developers and medical experts lay the technical groundwork, civil society is the bridge connecting this technology to the people it serves. By placing civil society at the heart of medical AI governance, we ensure that the technology serves humanity in the truest sense, governed by principles of ethics, equity, and empathy. As we move forward, let's champion a collaborative approach, ensuring that the future of medical AI is shaped by diverse voices, working in harmony for the collective good

Chapter 5

Implementation and Change Management

The incorporation of artificial intelligence (AI) in healthcare systems and practices has moved beyond futuristic concepts and is now a tangible reality. Healthcare institutions globally are harnessing AI technologies to enhance efficiency, improve decision-making, and foster innovative treatments and care strategies. However, the successful deployment of AI in healthcare is not automatic; it necessitates meticulous planning and an understanding of crucial success factors. This chapter delves into the critical facets of implementing AI in healthcare - a task that extends beyond mere technical deployment to encompass a comprehensive strategy for change management.

As we navigate this transformative era, it becomes increasingly clear that the integration of AI in healthcare is not merely a technological upgrade but a complex process that requires a careful orchestration of multiple elements. It involves aligning technology with human expertise, adapting existing workflows to new AI-driven methodologies, and managing the profound impact on the roles and responsibilities of healthcare professionals.

This chapter aims to serve as a comprehensive guide, offering insights into the multifaceted process of AI implementation in healthcare. We will explore the following key areas:

Strategic Planning for AI Integration: Understand the importance of developing a clear, strategic vision for AI adoption in healthcare settings. This includes assessing organizational readiness, setting realistic goals, and identifying potential challenges.

Build a Competent Team: Building a successful AI team requires a strategic approach that goes beyond technical expertise. By defining a clear vision and goals, assembling a multidisciplinary team, fostering a culture of learning and collaboration, implementing responsible AI practices, and regularly evaluating and iterating on your strategies, you can build a team that is capable of harnessing the power of AI to revolutionize healthcare.

Technology Deployment and Integration: Understand the technical aspects of AI implementation, the selection of appropriate AI solutions, integration with existing healthcare systems, and ensuring scalability and sustainability.

Change Management Principles: Apply principles of effective change management tailored to healthcare organizations. This includes strategies for managing resistance, fostering a culture of innovation, and ensuring a smooth transition for healthcare staff.

Training and Capacity Building: Uncover the importance of training healthcare professionals to work alongside AI tools. This includes developing new skill sets, understanding AI capabilities and limitations, and redefining roles in an AI-enhanced healthcare environment.

Ethical Considerations and Patient Engagement: consider the ethical implications of AI in healthcare, focusing on patient consent, data privacy, and algorithmic transparency. Also discuss strategies for engaging patients in this new era of AI-driven care.

Monitoring, Evaluation, and Continuous Improvement: Highlight the need for ongoing monitoring and evaluation to assess the impact of

AI implementation. This includes setting up metrics for success, gathering feedback, and continuously improving AI systems.

Have Response Plan: A response plan must be put in place to mitigate adverse impacts to customers and the company if an AI-related lapse occurs.

As we embark on this journey, it is crucial to recognize that the implementation of AI in healthcare is more than just a technological endeavor; it is a transformation that touches upon the very core of how healthcare is delivered and experienced. By embracing both the possibilities and the challenges, we can pave the way for a future where AI not only augments healthcare but also redefines it for the betterment of all.

Strategic Planning

Before implementing AI in healthcare, it is crucial to establish clear objectives. What specific healthcare challenges do you aim to address using AI? What opportunities within the healthcare sector are you seeking to leverage? Your AI strategy should be intricately aligned with the long-term goals of your healthcare organization or practice. See Chapter 2

For many healthcare leaders, it's surprising to learn that the investment in developing AI solutions cannot yield returns through the deployment of isolated, individual use cases, or even just a few. This underscores the importance of having an AI strategy that is cohesive and coordinated across the healthcare organization, in close alignment with its overarching healthcare strategy.

However, it's common for healthcare leaders to misorder the planning process, overly focusing on specific use cases or delegating the leadership of AI strategy to IT or data science departments. This approach can lead to a slippery slope, diminishing the organization's capacity to leverage AI for enhancing patient care, improving operational efficiency, advancing research, and more.

The most robust AI strategies in healthcare often start without directly focusing on AI. Instead, they begin with the organization's core strategy - its primary goals and objectives in healthcare. The process requires close collaboration with leaders across different departments and engagement of staff at all levels. The AI strategy should act as an enabler to the overall healthcare strategy, aligning with the same key performance indicators (KPIs) that are designed to enhance and grow the organization's competitive edge in healthcare.

Taking inspiration from a well-known example in the corporate world, a similar approach can be applied in healthcare. Leaders across the organization should be mandated to plan how they would use AI and machine learning (ML) to advance the organization's healthcare goals. This directive should drive innovation and can be a catalyst for establishing the organization as a leader in AI-powered healthcare.

These departmental plans should then be synthesized at the higher level, ensuring that mutual goals and initiatives are aligned with the core healthcare strategy. This step is crucial: only when AI is integrated across the entire healthcare organization can it deliver the combination of efficiency and value-creating outcomes necessary to sustain ongoing benefits and advancements in healthcare.

Build a Competent AI Team

AI in healthcare is a multidisciplinary field that requires a diverse set of skills and expertise. Your team should include:

Data Scientists and AI Specialists: These are the individuals who will develop and implement your AI models. They should have a strong background in machine learning, statistics, and programming.

Healthcare Professionals: Doctors, nurses, and other healthcare professionals can provide valuable insights into the healthcare problems you are trying to solve and can help ensure that your AI solutions are clinically relevant and useful.

Ethicists and Legal Experts: These individuals can guide your team in navigating the ethical and legal challenges associated with using AI in healthcare, such as issues related to patient privacy and data security.

Project Managers: Project managers can help coordinate your team's efforts, manage resources, and ensure that your AI projects stay on track and within budget.

Choosing the right AI technology

Successfully translating the potential of AI into reality requires careful consideration of the technical aspects involved in AI implementation. This includes the crucial steps of technology deployment and integration, encompassing the selection of appropriate AI solutions, seamless integration with existing healthcare systems, and ensuring scalability and sustainability for long-term success.

Selecting the Right AI Solutions:

The first step in AI implementation is selecting the appropriate AI solutions that align with the healthcare organization's goals and needs. This involves understanding the specific problems that need to be addressed, the available data, and the potential impact of different AI technologies. For instance, machine learning algorithms might be suitable for predicting patient outcomes based on historical data, while natural language processing could be used to analyze patient feedback or clinical notes.

Conducting a thorough analysis of existing workflows, data availability, and pain points is crucial for determining the most suitable AI solutions. This requires collaboration between healthcare professionals, data scientists, and technology experts to ensure the chosen AI solutions are clinically relevant, technically feasible, and address identified needs effectively.

The selection process also involves evaluating the technical feasibility and performance of different AI solutions. This includes considering factors such as the accuracy, speed, and robustness of the AI algorithms, as well as their ability to handle the complexity and variability of healthcare data.

Integrating AI with Existing Systems:

Once an appropriate AI solution has been selected, the next step is integrating it with the existing healthcare systems. This involves connecting the AI solution with the healthcare organization's data sources, workflows, and IT infrastructure.

Data integration is a key aspect of this process. Healthcare organizations typically have diverse data sources, including electronic health records, imaging systems, and laboratory information systems. The AI solution needs to be able to access and process this data in a secure and compliant manner.

Workflow integration is another important aspect. The AI solution should fit seamlessly into the healthcare professionals' workflows, enhancing their capabilities without adding unnecessary complexity or burden. This might involve integrating the AI solution with the healthcare organization's clinical decision support systems, patient management systems, or telemedicine platforms.

Ensuring Scalability and Sustainability

AI solutions need to be scalable to accommodate future growth and adapt to evolving healthcare needs. Building a modular architecture and leveraging cloud-based solutions can facilitate scalability and ensure efficient resource utilization. Additionally, establishing clear governance frameworks and monitoring systems is essential for controlling costs, preventing errors, and maintaining system reliability over time.

Technical Considerations:

Several technical aspects require careful attention during AI implementation:

Data Preparation and Management: Ensuring high-quality data with adequate volume and diversity is critical for training accurate and reliable AI models. Data cleaning, standardization, and anonymization are essential pre-processing steps, while robust data governance policies guarantee data security and compliance with ethical considerations.

Model Development and Training: Choosing appropriate algorithms and hyperparameter tuning are crucial for optimizing model performance. Explainability and interpretability of models are essential for healthcare professionals to understand and trust AI-driven insights.

Model Deployment and Monitoring: Deploying AI solutions in a production environment requires robust infrastructure and software engineering expertise. Continuous monitoring and evaluation are crucial for identifying and addressing model bias, performance degradation, and potential issues.

Navigating the Regulatory Landscape:

Understanding and adhering to relevant regulations governing patient data privacy, AI development, and clinical applications is crucial for ensuring ethical and legal compliance. Building compliance into the AI development lifecycle minimizes risks and ensures responsible implementation.

Engaging the public in discussions about AI in healthcare and actively contributing to policy development are essential for shaping a future where AI is used responsibly and ethically. Public understanding and support are crucial for ensuring AI serves the best interests of society.

Investing in ongoing training and development for healthcare professionals is critical for building the necessary skills and expertise to utilize AI effectively. Fostering a culture of collaboration and open communication between technical and healthcare professionals is essential for ensuring responsible AI development and deployment. Additionally, promoting ethical and regulatory compliance through robust frameworks and oversight mechanisms ensures that AI remains a force for good in healthcare.

Successfully deploying and integrating AI into healthcare requires a multifaceted approach that goes beyond the technology itself. By carefully selecting AI solutions, integrating them seamlessly with existing systems, ensuring scalability and sustainability, and addressing key technical considerations, we can pave the way for a future where AI empowers healthcare professionals to deliver better care and improve patient outcomes. By focusing on building a comprehensive and sustainable AI ecosystem, we can unlock the true potential of this transformative technology and create a healthier future for all.

Managing Change

Implementing responsible AI in healthcare, or any sector, is a transformative process that requires careful planning and execution. This includes key strategies for managing resistance, fostering a culture of innovation, and ensuring a smooth transition during the implementation of responsible AI.

Managing Resistance

Resistance to change is a natural human response. Resistance to change is a common phenomenon when introducing new technologies like AI. In the context of responsible AI, this resistance can stem from concerns about job security, patient safety, potential disruptions to workflows, ethical implications, or a lack of understanding about AI.

Effective strategies to manage resistance in AI implementation include:

Communication: Clearly communicate the ethical guidelines followed in the development and deployment of AI systems. Explain how responsible AI can enhance decision-making and efficiency, and address any misconceptions.

Involvement: Involve all stakeholders in the AI implementation process. This includes not only the technical team but also the end-users whose work will be directly impacted by the AI system.

Support: Provide training and resources to help stakeholders understand and adapt to the AI system. This could include training sessions on how the AI system works and how to interpret its outputs.

Fostering a Culture of Innovation

Innovation is crucial for the successful implementation of AI. Fostering a culture of innovation involves creating an environment where new ideas are encouraged, valued, and implemented. In the context of responsible AI, strategies to achieve this include:

Empowering Staff: Encourage staff to identify problems and propose solutions, creating opportunities for bottom-up innovation. This taps into the collective knowledge and expertise within the organization, leading to more effective and sustainable change.

Rewarding Innovation: Recognize and reward innovative ideas and practices that enhance the responsible use of AI.

Collaboration: Encourage collaboration between different teams to foster diverse perspectives and ideas. This can lead to more innovative and effective AI solutions.

Continuous Learning: Promote continuous learning and professional development to keep the team up-to-date with the latest developments in

AI and ethics. This can involve establishing innovation labs, sponsoring hackathons, and promoting cross-disciplinary collaboration.

Ensuring a Smooth Transition

Implementing AI can be disruptive, so it's important to ensure a smooth transition. This involves careful planning, ongoing support, and evaluation. Strategies to ensure a smooth transition include:

Phased Implementation: Implement the AI system in phases, allowing stakeholders to gradually adapt to the new system and provide feedback.

Change Champions: Identify and empower change champions who act as role models and support their colleagues throughout the transition. These individuals can provide guidance, address concerns, and help build enthusiasm for change.

Ongoing Support: Provide ongoing support during and after the AI implementation process. This can help stakeholders navigate challenges and feel supported.

Evaluation: Regularly evaluate the impact of the AI system to provide valuable feedback, demonstrate the benefits of the system, and guide future improvements.

Healthcare organizations face unique challenges due to the complex nature of their work and the critical importance of patient safety. Effective change management in healthcare requires tailoring strategies to these specific considerations. This includes:

Patient-Centric Approach: Ensure all changes are ultimately driven by the goal of improving patient care and outcomes. This maintains a clear focus and helps build consensus among stakeholders.

Data-Driven Decision Making: Utilize data and evidence to inform change decisions and track progress. This data-driven approach ensures changes are based on sound rationale and deliver measurable improvements.

Ethical Considerations: Carefully consider the ethical implications of any proposed change, ensuring patient data privacy, transparency in decision-making, and responsible use of technology.

Effectively navigating change in healthcare requires a holistic approach that addresses the emotional, technical, and organizational aspects of transformation. By adopting these tailored change management principles, healthcare organizations can foster a culture of innovation, manage resistance, and ensure a smooth and successful transition to new processes and technologies. Ultimately, implementing change effectively allows healthcare organizations to deliver better care, improve efficiency, and adapt to the ever-evolving landscape of healthcare delivery.

Training and Capacity Building

Realizing the full potential of this technology hinges on one crucial factor: the ability of healthcare professionals to effectively work alongside AI tools. This essay explores the importance of training and capacity building for healthcare professionals, emphasizing the development of new skill sets, understanding of AI capabilities and limitations, and redefining roles in an AI-enhanced healthcare environment.

Developing New Skill Sets:

Traditional healthcare curricula need to evolve to equip professionals with the necessary skills to thrive in an AI-driven environment. These skills include:

- Data literacy: Understanding how to interpret and analyze data generated by AI models, enabling healthcare professionals to critically evaluate their insights and make informed decisions.

- Technology competency: Familiarity with the basic principles of AI and the specific functionalities of the AI tools they utilize. This empowers them to interact with these tools effectively and troubleshoot any technical issues.
- Problem-solving and critical thinking: The ability to identify opportunities for AI integration, analyze complex data sets, and apply AI-driven insights to solve clinical challenges.

Understanding AI Capabilities and Limitations:

Unrealistic expectations surrounding AI can lead to misinterpretations and undermine its effectiveness. Healthcare professionals require training to understand:

- Strengths and limitations: AI tools excel at specific tasks, such as image recognition and pattern identification. However, they lack human understanding and nuance. Healthcare professionals need to be aware of these limitations to avoid overreliance and ensure AI complements, rather than replaces, their expertise.
- Bias and transparency: AI models can perpetuate societal biases present in training data. Understanding how to identify and mitigate bias is crucial for ensuring equitable and ethical application of AI in clinical settings.
- Accountability and responsibility: Ultimately, healthcare professionals remain accountable for patient care decisions. Training should emphasize the importance of critically evaluating AI outputs and maintaining human oversight to ensure patient safety and ethical considerations.

Redefining Roles and Responsibilities:

AI integration necessitates a reevaluation of traditional roles within healthcare. This may involve:

1. Collaborative teams: Healthcare professionals will increasingly work alongside AI specialists and data scientists, forming multidisciplinary teams that leverage each other's expertise.
2. Upskilling and reskilling: Some roles may evolve, requiring existing professionals to acquire new skills to adapt to the changing landscape.
3. New roles emerging: Specialized roles may emerge focused on managing AI systems, ensuring data quality, and developing new AI-driven healthcare solutions.

Building a Culture of Learning:

The rapid evolution of AI technologies necessitates a continuous learning culture within healthcare. This involves:

- Regular training and development programs: Providing ongoing updates on the latest advancements in AI and equipping healthcare professionals with the skills they need to stay current.
- Knowledge-sharing platforms: Creating platforms for healthcare professionals to share best practices, experiences, and challenges encountered while working with AI tools.
- Mentorship and support: Offering mentorship programs and support networks to help individuals navigate the changes and adapt to new roles and responsibilities.

Training and capacity building are not optional but essential for ensuring the successful integration of AI into healthcare. By equipping healthcare professionals with the necessary skills, knowledge, and understanding, we can unlock the full potential of this transformative technology. This will allow for human-AI collaboration to thrive, ultimately leading to improved patient care, greater efficiency, and a brighter future for healthcare.

Ethical Considerations and Patient Engagement

The implementation of Artificial Intelligence (AI) in healthcare raises critical ethical considerations, particularly concerning patient consent, data privacy, and algorithmic transparency. Balancing these ethical concerns with the benefits of AI is key to implementing responsible AI in healthcare.

The integration of AI in healthcare must navigate a complex ethical landscape. A primary concern is patient consent. Unlike traditional medical treatments, AI algorithms process vast amounts of patient data to make predictions or recommendations. Patients must be fully informed about how their data is used and the implications of AI-driven decisions on their care. Ensuring informed consent in this context requires clear communication about the capabilities and limitations of AI tools.

Engaging patients in AI-driven healthcare requires a multifaceted approach:

Educating Patients: Patients should be educated about the benefits and risks of AI in healthcare. This education should demystify AI technologies, providing patients with a clear understanding of how AI is used in their care and the safeguards in place to protect their data.

Enhancing Communication: AI can be leveraged to improve communication between patients and healthcare providers. For instance, AI-driven chatbots can provide patients with instant responses to queries, improving their engagement and satisfaction with healthcare services.

Co-design with Patients: Involving patients in the design and development of AI applications can ensure that these tools are attuned to their needs and concerns. This co-design approach can lead to more user-friendly and ethical AI solutions.

Transparency in AI Use: Patients should be informed when AI is being used as part of their diagnosis or treatment. Transparency about the role of AI in their care can build trust and acceptance among patients.

Feedback Mechanisms: Implementing mechanisms for patients to provide feedback on AI tools can help healthcare providers understand patient concerns and improve AI applications accordingly.

Promoting Patient Autonomy: AI should be used to augment, not replace, human decision-making in healthcare. Patients should have the option to discuss AI recommendations with their healthcare provider and make informed decisions about their care.

The ethical implementation of AI in healthcare is a balancing act between leveraging cutting-edge technology and respecting the rights and dignity of patients. Addressing concerns around patient consent, data privacy, and algorithmic transparency is essential for building trust and ensuring responsible use of AI. Moreover, actively engaging patients in this new era of AI-driven care is crucial for its success. By placing patients at the center of AI implementation strategies, healthcare providers can harness the full potential of AI while maintaining the highest ethical standards. Ultimately, the goal is not just to introduce advanced technology into healthcare, but to do so in a way that is aligned with the core values of medical practice: empathy, respect, and a commitment to patient well-being.

Monitoring and Evaluation

The successful implementation of Artificial Intelligence (AI) in healthcare requires more than simply deploying AI tools. To truly realize the potential of AI for improving patient care and optimizing healthcare delivery, a continuous cycle of monitoring, evaluation, and improvement is essential.

AI systems are not static entities. As technology evolves and healthcare needs change, AI systems need to be continuously monitored and evaluated to ensure they remain effective, ethical, and aligned with patient needs. This process serves several key purposes:

- Assessing impact: Measuring the impact of AI on key performance indicators (KPIs) such as patient outcomes, efficiency, and cost savings provides valuable insights into its effectiveness.
- Identifying bias and error: Monitoring and evaluation can reveal potential biases or errors in AI models, enabling timely intervention and corrective action.
- Ensuring compliance: Evaluating AI systems for compliance with ethical guidelines and regulatory requirements is crucial for ensuring responsible AI implementation.
- Promoting continuous improvement: Feedback from monitoring and evaluation activities provides vital information for improving AI models, algorithms, and workflows, leading to better patient care and outcomes.

Defining clear and measurable metrics is crucial for effectively monitoring and evaluating the impact of AI in healthcare. These metrics should be specific, quantifiable, achievable, relevant, and time-bound (SMART) and aligned with the desired goals of AI implementation. Examples of relevant metrics include:

- Patient outcomes: Improved diagnostics, reduced readmission rates, increased survival rates.
- Efficiency: Reduced time to diagnosis, faster treatment initiation, improved workflow optimization.
- Cost-effectiveness: Cost savings associated with AI-driven interventions, improved resource utilization.
- Patient satisfaction: Increased patient satisfaction with care, improved communication and understanding of AI-driven decisions.

Understanding the experiences and perspectives of patients, healthcare professionals, and other stakeholders is critical for comprehensive evaluation. Feedback can be gathered through various channels, including:

- Patient surveys and focus groups: Gaining patient insights into their understanding of AI, their experience with AI-driven care, and their level of trust.
- Staff surveys and interviews: Collecting feedback from healthcare professionals on their experiences using AI tools, identifying challenges and areas for improvement.
- Technical and Data analysis: Regular technical audits of AI systems help in identifying technical issues, data biases, or inefficiencies. Analyzing usage data, error logs, and other system-generated information to identify patterns and areas for improvement.

Monitoring and evaluation findings must be translated into concrete actions for continuous improvement. This may involve:

Updating AI models: Refining algorithms and training data to address identified biases, errors, and improve performance.

- Enhancing user interfaces and workflows: Making AI tools more user-friendly and accessible for healthcare professionals to ensure efficient integration into existing workflows.
- Adapting to Clinical Variabilities: Healthcare is subject to constant changes, including new medical discoveries and varying patient demographics. AI systems need regular updates to remain relevant and effective in this changing environment.
- Developing ethical frameworks and guidelines: Establishing clear guidelines and oversight mechanisms to govern the development and use of AI in healthcare, ensuring ethical and responsible implementation.
- Compliance with Regulatory Standards: Healthcare is a highly regulated field. Continuous evaluation ensures that AI systems

remain compliant with evolving regulatory requirements, such as those related to patient privacy and data security.
- Educating and training healthcare professionals: Providing healthcare professionals with the knowledge and skills needed to effectively utilize AI tools and understand their limitations.

Monitoring, evaluation, and continuous improvement form the cornerstone of responsible AI implementation in healthcare. By establishing clear metrics, actively seeking feedback, and implementing ongoing improvement strategies, we can ensure that AI serves as a powerful tool for enhancing patient care, advancing healthcare delivery, and ultimately, creating a healthier future for all.

Build a Response Plan

In the context of healthcare, the establishment and testing of a response plan are fundamental to operationalizing Responsible AI. While proactive measures are essential to prevent lapses in AI applications, healthcare organizations must also recognize that errors can occur. Consequently, a well-structured response plan is necessary to mitigate any adverse impacts on patients and the healthcare institution if an AI-related lapse happens. This plan should outline clear steps to prevent further harm, address technical issues promptly, and communicate transparently with patients, healthcare professionals, and stakeholders about the nature of the issue and the corrective actions being taken.

It is crucial that the response plan specifies the individuals responsible for each action, ensuring clarity and efficient execution during a crisis. This delineation of responsibilities is vital to avoid confusion and to guarantee that response measures are implemented swiftly and effectively.

Developing, validating, testing, and refining procedures are essential to ensure that in the event of an AI system failure, negative consequences are minimized as much as possible. In healthcare, where patient safety and wellbeing are paramount, the stakes are particularly high.

One effective way to evaluate the robustness of this response plan is through a tabletop exercise that simulates an AI lapse. This simulated scenario is an invaluable tool for healthcare executives and teams to assess the organization's preparedness and identify any existing gaps in the response strategy. This approach, akin to methods used in cybersecurity, allows healthcare leaders to experience firsthand how the organization would react to an AI-related incident, thereby enhancing the overall effectiveness of the response plan.

In summary, crafting a thorough and actionable response plan is a critical aspect of implementing Responsible AI in healthcare. It ensures that healthcare organizations are not only prepared to prevent AI lapses but are also equipped to handle them effectively should they occur, thereby safeguarding patient welfare and maintaining the integrity of healthcare services.

Bringing it all together

The development and implementation of AI in healthcare is complex and costly, so health organizations need to make smart decisions and develop strategic plans that enable them to bring real value to their organizations. Below are some considerations for the successful development, deployment, and integration of AI in healthcare.

Considering both short-term and long-term goals of your organization

As decision-makers, it is essential to consider both the shortterm and long-term goals when you develop an AI strategy for your organization. In the short term, you need to build a use case by identifying the most pressing problems that your organization is facing and determine how such problems can be solved by cost-effective AI technologies and methods available. In the long term, you need to envision the future of your organization, considering how your organization may evolve and how the existing and emerging AI technologies can be scaled to effectively transform your organization, building a hospital of tomorrow.

Many health organizations are currently focused on ML on hospital EHR data. As the 5G super-fast connectivity becomes available, there will be a convergence of technologies of AI, sensors, voice chatbots, virtual/augmented reality, and other interactive media. Real-time monitoring, diagnoses, and treatment optimization based on historical and current data of both individuals and the population will become possible. This will allow the development of an intelligent, integrated, and connected nationwide digital health ecosystem that will not only support medical decision-making and clinical research but will also improve patient education, participation, and are at home. So, health leaders need to design their AI strategies and infrastructure capacities with a view on both the present and the future.

Establishing the leadership, team, culture, and collaboration for successful implementation

Technology alone will not transform healthcare; it needs people who derive value from AI and who create impact across your organization. Senior leaders can make a difference in their AI projects by providing the funding, talent, and resources required. In addition, it is crucial to build a team of people who possess the diverse expertise required for AI development, technology integration, data migration, and medical service integrations. It is equally important to develop a corporate culture for organization-wide participation in AI innovation. Health organizations should be prepared to collaborate with partners across the industry, working with partners to make smart decisions and bring the AI implementation and integration to success.

Selecting the right AI platform, tools, and approaches for implementing your AI strategy

Healthcare providers vary in their sizes, types, challenges, priorities, and resources. For providers that have already installed a sound EHR system, adding AI capabilities into the EHR system is possible as many EHR vendors have opened their platforms to allow data exchange and system connection. In addition, many vendors are adding AI features into their EHR systems. For most hospitals, working with the HER vendor and other AI technology firm to develop the solutions they need is perhaps the best option. For organizations that have the expertise and resources to build their own AI capabilities or that want to become an AI player in the healthcare industry, they can do so by using commercial AI cloud platforms and services currently available. To keep business as usual, they can build their new AI infrastructure and process independently, then link it to the old infrastructure. This gives health organizations complete control in instantiating a new process while avoiding interfering with the ongoing operations.

Forming a good data strategy to derive patient insights

Successful ML relies on the access to large volumes of quality data; the source, size, and quality of data can dramatically impact the ML models developed. Collecting large-scale data that are complete, accurate, up-to-date, and representative of typical populations is a big challenge for analytics professionals. Part of the bias in AI is due to the lack of diverse data available for training the algorithms. So the capacity to collect, store, and learn from data is crucial for AI success and often AI workers spend a large part of theirtime to clean up data in order to ensure the quality of the ML models they are developing. Some data scientists believe that collecting new data that meet the current data standards is better than cleaning up old messy data. This is a valid perspective because the old data in EHR systems often contain noises, biases, errors, and unusable data.

Retraining ML algorithms and validating AI applications with data and patients from the local organizations

Not including enough meaningful and representative data during training and validation is a common problem in ML. Health organizations need to understand such limitations and provide adequate, balanced, diverse, and representative data from its population for retraining and validating ML models when they deploy them. Decision-makers need to be aware that most AI technologies are not "out-of-the-box" products that you can simply plug into your digital system for it to work. Small-scale on-site pilot testing is a good way to validate any AI application

Determining the context and protocols for the safe use of AI technology

Ensuring the safety, privacy, and well-being of patients requires one to conduct a hazard analysis, evaluate the consequences of potential false positive and false negative, and develop hazard prevention protocols. For crucial clinical processes that can lead to serious consequences (eg, making medical diagnosis and treatment decisions), a dual safety mechanism is required. In such cases, doctors are the ones who make the calls, using data-generated insights as references. Furthermore, for any AI product to be deployed, an on-site pilot implementation and validation is needed. Finally, it is important to collect realworld evidence and develop a mechanism to continuously monitor system performance, ensuring the safety and effectiveness of the deployed AI product on an ongoing basis. In all these processes, it is important to establish policies and protocols to ensure the privacy, security, and ethics of AI use. However, we must keep a balance between patient privacy and data sharing, and between regulation and innovation. Artificial intelligence professionals need to work with a large volume of real patient data to ensure the accuracy and safety of the ML models, so patients need to know that AI can only be advanced when they share data more freely, and this can be done in a secure environment. Meanwhile, health organizations need to ensure that their AI approaches are lawful, ethical, and robust, showing complete transparency about what they do with patient data.

Establishing performance standards to measure AI success

Assessing AI approaches takes time but it will enable health organizations to discover problems and fix them before it is too late. Before implementation, it is essential to define performance evaluation metrics, then measure

AI success accordingly at different stages of the development and implementation (eg, pilot testing, scaled implementation, and validation). Such performance metrics should reflect the values, priorities, and vision of your organization. There are many ways to assess AI technologies. Generally speaking, things to consider in the evaluation should include improved clinical effectiveness (quality, efficiency, and safety), extended access and expanded services to patients, improved patient experience and outcomes, optimized operational processes, improved staff satisfaction with the work environment, and reduced costs and increased revenue

Chapter 6

AI Risks, Risk Assessment and Risk Mitigation

While AI promises groundbreaking advances in patient care and healthcare management, it also brings forth a spectrum of risks that must be carefully navigated. This chapter delves into the critical risks associated with the integration of AI in healthcare, aiming to provide a comprehensive understanding of these challenges and the strategies required for effective risk mitigation.

We identify and analyze seven key categories of risks that have emerged as significant concerns in the literature and practice:

1. Patient harm due to AI errors
2. Misuse of medical AI tools
3. Risk of bias in medical AI and perpetuation of inequities
4. Lack of transparency
5. Privacy and security issues
6. Gaps in AI accountability
7. Obstacles to implementation in real-world healthcare

Not only could these risks result in harms for the patients and citizens, but they could also reduce the level of trust in AI algorithms on the part of clinicians and society at large. Hence, risk assessment, classification and management must be an integral part of the AI development, evaluation and deployment processes.

Patient harm due to AI errors

Despite continuous advances in data availability and machine learning, AI-guided clinical solutions in healthcare may be associated with failures that could potentially result in safety concerns for the end-users of healthcare services. These AI algorithm errors can lead, for example, to (1) false negatives in the form of missed diagnoses of life-threatening diseases, (2) unnecessary treatments due to false positives (healthy persons incorrectly classified as diseased by the AI algorithm), (3) unsuitable interventions due to imprecise diagnosis, or incorrect prioritization of interventions in emergency departments.

Assuming that AI developers have access to large-scale datasets with sufficient quality for training their AI technologies, there are still at least three major sources of error for AI in clinical practice. Firstly, AI predictions can be significantly impacted by noise in the input data during the usage of the AI tool. For example, ultrasound scanning – the most commonly used imaging modality in clinical practice due to its low-cost and portability – is known to be prone to scanning errors This depends particularly on the experience of the operator, the cooperation of the patient, and the clinical context (e.g. emergency ultrasound). Even in high-income countries where there is a high level of medical training, such errors are expected to occur in some scans, thus affecting subsequent AI predictions.

Secondly, AI misclassifications may appear due to dataset shift, a common problem in machine learning that occurs when the statistical distribution of the data used in clinical practice is shifted, even slightly, from the original distribution of the dataset used to train the AI algorithm. This shift could be due to differences in the population groups, acquisition protocols between hospitals, or the usage of machines from different manufacturers. A recent study has shown that AI models trained on cardiac magnetic resonance image (MRI) scans from two scanners (e.g. Siemens and Philips) lose accuracy when applied to MRI data acquired from different machines (e.g. General Electric and Canon).

Another example of dataset shift can be seen in a multi-center study in the United States that built a highly accurate pneumonia diagnosis AI system based on data from two hospitals. When tested with data from a third hospital, a significant decrease in accuracy was noticed, suggesting potential hospital-specific biases. In another example, the company DeepMind developed a deep learning model trained on a large dataset for automated diagnosis of retinal diseases from optical coherence tomography (OCT). They found that the AI system was confused when applied to images obtained from a machine that is different from the one used for data acquisition at the AI training stage, with the diagnosis error increasing from 5.5% to a staggering 46%. These examples illustrate the current challenges posed in building AI tools that maintain a high level of accuracy even if the data is heterogeneous across populations, hospitals or machines.

Lastly, the predictions can be erroneous due to the difficulty of AI algorithms to adapt to unexpected changes in the environment and context in which they are applied. To illustrate the problem, researchers at Harvard Medical School described a nice example in the domain of AI for medical imaging. They imagined an AI system that was trained to detect shadows or dense features on a chest X-ray images that are associated with lesions in major diseases such as lung cancer. Then, they listed a number of simple scenarios in which the AI may lead to incorrect predictions, such as if the X-ray technician leaves the adhesive ECG connectors on their patient's chest or if the patient wears a wedding ring and places their hand on their chest during the scan. In these scenarios, it is possible that the AI model could mistake these circular artefacts as one of the known chest lesions, resulting in a false positive.

There are at least three avenues to minimize the risk of AI errors and safety issues for patients). First of all, standardized methods and procedures need to be defined for extensive evaluation and regulatory approval of AI solutions, in particular regarding their generalizability to new populations and sensitivity to noise. Second, the AI algorithms should be designed and implemented as assistive tools (as opposed to fully autonomous tools), such that clinicians remain part of the data processing workflow to detect and report potential errors and contextual changes, and hence to minimise harm to patients.

Furthermore, future AI solutions in healthcare must be dynamic, i.e., they should be embedded with mechanisms to continue to learn from new scenarios and mistakes as they are detected in practice. However, this last aspect will still require a certain degree of human control and vigilance to identify problems as they appear; this in turn may increase costs and reduce the initial benefits of AI. Infrastructural and technical developments will also be needed to enable regular AI updates (based on past and new training), and it will be necessary to implement policies that ensure such mechanisms are integrated into healthcare settings.

CAUSES OF AI ERRORS	MEDICAL CONSEQUENCES	MITIGATION MEASURES
• Noise and artefacts in AI's clinical inputs and measurements • Data shift between AI training data and real-world data • Unexpected variations in clinical contexts and environments	• Missed diagnosis of life-threatening conditions • False diagnosis and thus inadequate treatments • Incorrect scheduling or prioritisation of interventions	1. Comprehensive multi-centre evaluation studies to identify instabilities 2. Assistive AI solutions that maintain the clinician as part of the workflow 3. Traceable and dynamic AI solutions that continue to improve over time

Misuse of Medical AI tools

As with most health technologies, there is a risk for human error and human misuse with medical AI. Even when the developed AI algorithms are accurate and robust, they are dependent on the way they are used in practice by the end-users, including clinicians, healthcare professionals, and patients. Incorrect usage of AI tools can result in incorrect medical assessment and decision making and subsequently in potential harm for the patient. Hence, it is not enough for clinicians and the general public to have access to medical AI tools, but it is also necessary for them to understand how and when to use these technologies.

There are multiple factors that make existing medical AI technologies prone to human error or incorrect use. First, they have often been designed and developed by computer/data scientists with limited involvement from end-users and clinical experts. As a result, it is the user (i.e., the clinician, the nurse, the data manager or the patient) that is required to learn to use and to adapt to the new AI technology, which can lead to unnatural and complex interactions and experiences. In turn, the clinical user may encounter difficulties in understanding and applying the AI algorithm in day-to-day practice, which will limit the perception of informed decision making, while increasing the chances of human error.

This problem is exacerbated by the fact that existing training programs in medicine are not yet tailored for medical AI and generally do not equip new clinicians with knowledge and skills in the area of AI. In 2021, a significant number of medical trainees in Australia and New Zealand across various specialties like ophthalmology, dermatology, and oncology expressed optimism about AI improving their fields, particularly in enhancing disease screening and simplifying repetitive tasks. Despite this positive outlook, a vast majority of these trainees had not used AI in their clinical practice, and only a small fraction felt they had an excellent understanding of AI.

Similarly, medical students in the UK faced a gap in AI education, with many reporting that their curriculum did not include compulsory AI training. This trend was not limited to the UK; healthcare professionals across the European Union also showed limited familiarity with and usage of technology-based interventions in healthcare.

This lack of AI literacy is also evident among the general public. Surveys across several countries, including Australia, the US, Canada, Germany, and the UK, revealed that public awareness and understanding of AI, especially in its application to daily life, were generally low. While certain demographics, such as younger individuals, men, and university-educated groups, had slightly better awareness, their overall understanding of AI was still only modest at best.

Another cause for potential misuse of medical AI, which could lead to harm for citizens and patients, is the proliferation of easily accessible medical AI applications. For example, commercial mobile apps have been developed by several companies for skin cancer detection with the purpose of enabling individuals to take and upload a picture of their skin through the app, which is then directly analysed and assessed by the app's AI algorithm. Some examples of such apps include Skinvision, MelApp, skinScan and SpotMole.

While these tools are easily accessible to the general public, there is often limited information on how the AI algorithms in question have been developed and validated, while their reliability and clinical efficacy is not always demonstrated. For example, a recent study which evaluated six mobile apps for skin cancer detection demonstrated their lack of efficiency and high risk for bias The authors concluded: 'Current algorithm-based smartphone apps cannot be relied on to detect all cases of melanoma or other skin cancers. The current regulatory process for awarding the CE marking for algorithm-based apps does not provide adequate protection to the public'.

A quick search shows that many AI-powered online/mobile tools have also emerged in a wide range of medical domains and are commercially offered for medical diagnostics and health monitoring. While such services can constitute a promising solution for remote diagnosis and disease follow-up, their wide proliferation online can become a public health concern, in the same way that easily accessible online pharmacies have contributed to an abuse of medication by citizens.

Since there is a lot of financial gain to be made from the development and commercialization of AI-powered web/mobile health applications, this sector will continue to attract a lot of new players and companies with varying standards of ethics, excellence and quality. The companies offering these web or mobile based AI medical tools acknowledge on their websites that their AI products are not certified medical devices and the terms of service often contain disclaimers. One can easily find disclaimers such as 'this site is designed to offer you general health information for educational purposes only' or 'the health information furnished on this site and the interactive responses are not intended to be professional advice and are not intended to replace personal consultation with a qualified physician, pharmacist or other healthcare professional'. However, most users may not necessarily come across, read and comprehend these disclaimers, and hence may rely on potentially incorrect information and diagnoses provided by the AI tools, which may negatively impact their decision making regarding their health.

There are several avenues to reduce human error or incorrect use of future medical AI solutions. First of all, end-users such as healthcare professionals, specialists, technicians or patients should be closely involved in the design and development of AI solutions to ensure their points of view, preferences and contexts are well integrated into the final tools that will be deployed and used. Furthermore, education and literacy programmes on AI and medical AI should be developed and generalised across education circles and society to increase the knowledge and skills of future AI end-users and hence reduce human error. Finally, it is important that public agencies help regulate the sector of web/mobile medical AI, such that the citizens are well informed and protected against the misuse and abuse of these emerging, easily accessible AI technologies.

POTENTIAL CAUSES OF AI MISUSE

1. Limited involvement of clinicians and citizens in AI developments
2. Lack of AI training in medical AI among healthcare professionals
3. Lack of awareness and literacy among patients and the general public
4. Proliferation of easily accessible online and mobile AI solutions

MITIGATION MEASURES

1. User-centred design and extensive usability tests for the AI algorithms
2. Future integration of AI education and training in medical schools
3. New literacy programmes to increase medical AI knowledge in society
4. Better regulation and information on emerging AI technologies

Risk of bias in medical AI and perpetuation of inequities

Despite continuous advances in medical research and healthcare delivery, there remain important inequalities and inequities in medical care within most countries around the world. The main factors that contribute to these inequalities and inequities include sex/gender, age, ethnicity, income, education and geography. While some of these inequities are systemic, such as due to socioeconomic differences and discrimination, human biases also play an important role. For example, in the United States, existing research has demonstrated that doctors do not take Black patients' complaints of pain as seriously nor do they respond to them as quickly as they do for their White counterparts. Persistent in most countries around the world, to varying degrees, is yet another example of common bias embedded in healthcare systems: gender-based discrimination. Once again, in the domain of pain management, studies have pointed to the increased psychologization or invisibilisation of female patients when reporting pain.

Hence, in the recent years, there have been concerns that, if not properly implemented, evaluated and regulated, future AI solutions could embed and even amplify the systemic disparities and human biases that contribute to healthcare inequities. A few examples of algorithmic biases have already made the headlines in recent years, some of which are detailed below.

A study published in Science in 2019 showed that an algorithm used in the United States to help in the referral process of patients who need extra or specialist care was shown to discriminate against Black patients. The authors of the study explained that with the algorithm, 'at a given risk score, Black patients are considerably sicker than White patients, as evidenced by signs of uncontrolled illnesses. Remedying this disparity would increase the percentage of Black patients receiving additional help from 17.7 to 46.5%'. A Canadian study in 2020 evaluated the degree of fairness of state-of-the-art deep learning algorithms used to detect abnormalities such as fractures, lung lesions, nodules, pneumonia, etc. in chest X-ray images. The study showed that the highest rate of underdiagnosis was in young females (age: 0-20), in Black patients, and in patients on public health insurance for low-income people and households. Furthermore, patients with intersectional identities (for example, a Hispanic female patient on low- income health insurance) suffered the highest rates of underdiagnosis. The authors concluded that 'models trained on large datasets do not provide equality of opportunity naturally, leading instead to potential disparities in care if deployed without modification.

It is widely argued that the most common cause for unfairness in medical AI is the bias in the data used to train the machine learning models. Bias is already part of the clinical landscape. So, it is not as if machine learning is out to get us. It is that when we are training on data that humans make, that humans label, that humans annotate, we might pick up on some of the biases that humans have injected into that data.

As an example, in 2002 the National Lung Screening Trial, which compiled datasets from 53,000 smokers to investigate methods for early diagnosis of lung cancer, was found to include only 4% of Black participants in the data. Machine learning algorithms for skin cancer detection have been all-too-often trained on highly biased datasets – such as the International Skin Imaging Collaboration, one of the most widely used open-access database of skin lesions – which contain images from mostly fair-skinned patients in the United States, Europe, and Australia. Diagnostic models only trained on fair-skin groups could prove to be detrimental to the diagnostic process of melanoma lesions present on dark-skinned individuals. Similarly, the way COVID-19 appears to affect patients differently according to their sex group means an AI algorithm trained on existing clinical data is likely to suffer from reduced fairness when predicting severity and mortality in men and women.

Another type of bias that appears in datasets is of a geographic nature. In 2020, researchers from the fields of radiology and biomedical research at Stanford University conducted a review of articles published over a five-year period that had been used in training deep learning algorithms related to patient care. They found that 71% of the United States studies in which geographic location was identified used data only from California, Massachusetts, and New York. In addition, they found the studies did not include any data from 34 of the 50 states in the U.S. Geographic bias can be an important issue in Europe too, as data availability and access to digital equipment are unevenly distributed, particularly in the Eastern European regions.

Another potential source of lack of fairness in medical AI is bias in the data labelling during clinical assessment. For example, existing research has shown that due to gender stereotypes, women are over-diagnosed for some diseases such as depression and under-diagnosed for other diseases such as cancer. Furthermore, a large-scale Danish study, which analyzed data on hospital admissions for approximately 7 million citizens and 19 disease groups, found that for the vast majority of the diseases, women are diagnosed later than men. Importantly, for many of these medical conditions such as injury, poisoning, congenital malformations and infectious diseases, these discrepancies cannot be explained by anatomical or genetic differences. If the data labels in the health registries are affected by such healthcare disparities, such as in environments where given groups have been systematically misdiagnosed due to stigma or stereotypes, then the AI models will likely learn to perpetuate this disparity.

In recent years, awareness of algorithmic bias has increased and researchers, particularly in North America, have started to investigate mitigation measures to address the risk of unfairness in medical AI. First, it is evident that AI developers, in collaboration with clinical experts and healthcare professionals, must pay close and continuous attention to the selection and labelling of the data and variables to be used during model training. These should be representative and balanced with respect to key attributes such as sex/gender, age, socioeconomics, ethnicity, as well as geographic location. Furthermore, it is recommended to involve not only data scientists and biomedical researchers in the development teams, but also social scientists, biomedical ethicists, public health experts, as well as patients and citizens. The latter group must be as diverse as possible to ensure that adequate diversity of backgrounds, experiences and needs are taken into consideration during the AI production lifecycle and that the tools created are truly representative and founded on community-based research.

MOST COMMON BIASES IN MEDICAL AI	MOST COMMON CAUSES OF AI BIASES	MITIGATION MEASURES
· According to sex and gender · According to age differences · According to ethnic groups · According to geographic locations · According to socioeconomics	· Biased and imbalanced datasets · Structural biases and discrimination · Disparities in access to quality equipment and digital technologies · Lack of diversity and interdisciplinarity in development teams	1. Systemic AI training with balanced, representative datasets 2. Interdisciplinary approaches in medical AI involving social scientists 3. Promotion of more diversity and inclusion in the field of medical AI

Lack of transparency

Despite continuous advances in medical AI, existing algorithms continue to be viewed by individuals and experts alike as complex and obscure technologies, which are difficult to fully comprehend, trust and adopt.

A recent AI algorithm developed by Google for breast cancer screening received considerable attention for its promising performance. It was shown to improve the speed and robustness of breast cancer screening, to generalize well to populations in multiple countries beyond those used for training, and it even outperformed radiologists in specific situations. However, this work also received some criticism in the media and in the AI community as it was presented with almost no details on how the algorithm was built and on key technical descriptions. Some critics questioned the usefulness and safety of such an AI tool, while a group of scientists used this algorithm as their central example when they published a call in Nature for more transparency in medical AI.

Lack of transparency is widely regarded as an important issue in the development and use of current AI tools in healthcare. It is expected to result in a great lack of trustworthiness in AI especially in sensitive areas such as medicine and healthcare that are focused on the wellbeing and health of citizens. At the same time, a lack of trustworthiness will evidently impact the level of adoption of emerging AI algorithms by patients, clinicians, and healthcare systems.

AI transparency is closely linked to the concepts of traceability and explainability, which correspond to two distinct levels at which transparency is required, i.e. (1) transparency of the AI development and usage processes (traceability), and (2) transparency of the AI decisions (explainability).

Traceability is considered a key requirement for trustworthy AI, and refers to transparently documenting the whole AI development process, including tracking how the AI model functions in real-world practice after deployment. More specifically, traceability requires maintaining a complete account of (i) model details (intended use, type of algorithm or neural network, hyper-parameters, as well as pre- and post-processing steps),

(ii) training and validation data (gathering process, data composition, acquisition protocols and data labelling) and

(iii) AI tool monitoring (performance metrics, failures, periodic evaluations)

In practice, existing AI tools in healthcare are rarely delivered with full traceability. In fact, companies often prefer not to disclose too much information about their algorithms, which are thus delivered as opaque tools that are difficult to understand and examine by independent parties. This, in turn, reduces the level of trust and adoption into real-world practice.

While traceability addresses the transparency of the AI algorithm's lifecycle, AI explainability is important for providing transparency for each AI prediction and decision. Article 22 of the European Union's General Data Protection Regulation (GDPR) details the 'right to explanation' which requires an explanation to be offered regarding the automated decision-making process.

However, AI solutions, and specifically deep neural networks lack transparency, and are often described as 'black box AI', referring to the fact that these models learn complex functions that humans struggle to understand and whose functions and decision-making processes are not visible or understandable. A lack of transparency makes it difficult for clinicians and other stakeholders to incorporate AI solutions into their real-world practice because in order to work with specific AI solutions, clinicians need to be able to understand the fundamental principles behind each decision and/or prediction, even when the algorithm itself has the potential to enhance the clinician's productivity. Furthermore, the lack of explainability means that it is difficult to identify the source of AI errors and define responsibilities when it goes wrong.

There are numerous avenues available to improve the transparency of AI technologies in healthcare. First of all, there is a need for an 'AI passport' that could be a requirement for each AI algorithm for documenting all the model's key information. There is also a need to develop traceability tools for monitoring the usage of AI algorithms once they are deployed, such as to record potential errors and performance degradation, as well as to perform periodic audits. To improve the explainability of AI algorithms, it is important that AI developers involve clinical end-users from the start of the development process in order to select the best explainability approach for each application and to ensure that the chosen explanations are useful and well accepted in clinical practice. Finally, regulatory entities can play an important role by considering the traceability and explainability of the AI tools as pre-requisites for certification.

RISKS ASSOCIATED WITH LACK OF TRANSPARENCY IN MEDICAL AI

1. Lack of understanding and trust in AI predictions and decisions
2. Difficulties to independently reproduce and evaluate AI algorithms
3. Difficulties to identify the sources of AI errors and define responsibilities
4. Limited uptake of AI tools in clinical practice and the real world

MITIGATION MEASURES

1. Create an AI passport for documenting all the model's key information
2. Create a traceability tool to monitor the usage of AI algorithms
3. Involve clinical end-users in the design of clinically explainable AI tools
4. Include traceability and explainability as prerequisites for certification

MAIN DETAILS
- Identifier:
- Owner(s):
- TRL level:
- Licence:
- Data of creation:

INTENDED USE
- Primary use:
- Secondary use:
- Users:
- Counter-indications:
- Ethical considerations:

MODEL DETAILS
- Model design:
- Model hyperparameters:
- Objective functions:
- Fairness constraints:

TRAINING DATA
- Data provenance:
- Population groups:
- Variables:
- Pre-processing

EVALUATION
- Evaluation data:
- Evaluation metrics:
- Evaluation results:
- Identified limitations:

MONITORING
- Last periodic evaluation:
- Identified failures:
- Version number:

MISCELLANEOUS
- Assumptions:

AI Passport

Privacy and security issues

The increasingly widespread development of AI solutions and technology in healthcare, recently highlighted by the COVID-19 pandemic, has shown potential risks for a lack of data privacy, confidentiality and protection for patients and citizens. This could lead to serious consequences, such as the exposure and use of sensitive data which goes against the rights of the citizens or the repurposing of patient data for non-medical gains.

These issues are firstly linked to informed consent, i.e., the provision of adequate information for the patients for an informed decision such as for sharing personal health data. Informed consent is a crucial and integral part to the patient's experience in healthcare, which was formalized in the Helsinki Declaration and has since grown as the introduction of digital technology has permeated our daily lives. Informed consent is linked to various ethical issues, including protection from harm, respect for autonomy, privacy protection and property rights concerning data and/or tissue.

However, the introduction of opaque AI algorithms and complicated informed consent forms limits the level of autonomy and the power of shared patient-physician decision making. It has become increasingly difficult for patients to understand the decision-making process and the different ways in which their data can be reused, and to know exactly how they can choose to opt out of sharing their data. Issues of informed consent are also especially prominent in big data research, especially digital platform-based health data research, in which a patient may not be fully aware of or fully understand the extent to which their data is shared and reused.

An important example of this occurred in 2016, when records of 1.6 million patients in the United Kingdom were transferred – without patients' informed consent – from the Royal Free NHS Foundation Trust to the Google-owned AI company DeepMind, which at the time was working on developing an app to implement new ways of detecting kidney disease. In

July 2017, the UK Information Commissioner's Office (ICO) ruled that the Royal Free NHS Trust had breached data protection laws; the Information Commissioner office was famously quoted as saying, 'the price of innovation does not need to be the erosion of fundamental privacy rights'.

The use of AI in healthcare also entails a risk of data security breaches, in which personal information may be made widely available, infringing on citizens' rights to privacy and putting them at risk for identity theft and other types of cyberattacks. In July 2020, the New York based AI company Cense AI suffered a data breach that exposed highly sensitive data of upwards of 2.5 million patients who had suffered from car accidents, including such detailed information as names, addresses diagnostic notes, dates and types of accident, insurance policy numbers and more. Although eventually secured, this data was briefly accessible to anyone in the world with an internet connection, underlining the very real danger of personal privacy breaches that patients are exposed to.

Another persistent concern is that of data repurposing, which in certain contexts is also referred to as 'function creep'. The World Health Organization has warned against the danger of function creep during the COVID-19 pandemic, highlighting a case in Singapore in which the data from the government's COVID-19 tracing applications was also made available for criminal investigations. This is a stark example of health-related data being repurposed for non-healthcare related ends, but repurposing can also occur within the healthcare sphere itself. Data from electronic health records, registry data and data from health systems are used for pharmaceutical drug development, clinical trial design, marketing and cost-effectiveness analyses, and more.

In addition to the issues related to data privacy and security, AI tools are especially vulnerable to cyberattacks, the results of which could be anything from burdensome to fatal, depending on the context. In September 2020, a patient died after having to be redirected to another hospital when the Düsseldorf University Hospital suffered a cyberattack that interfered with the hospital's data and rendered the center's computer system inoperable.

Although it was later argued that it could not be proven that the death was directly caused by the cyberattack, because the patient was already suffering a life-threatening condition, this case brought to the forefront the real physical harms that cyberattacks can cause in the healthcare sphere.

In another example of how technological breaches may affect the physical health of patients, in April 2021 the Swedish oncology software company Elekta suffered a healthcare ransomware attack that affected 170 health systems in the United States, delaying cancer treatment care to patients across the country as well as exposing sensitive patient data.

Furthermore, research has shown that personal medical devices controlled by AI are also vulnerable to attacks. For example, researchers discovered that AI-powered insulin pumps for diabetes patients could be hacked and remotely controlled from varying distances, and could even be manipulated to flood the patient's body with excessive insulin). While this hack has never been carried out in the real world, researchers' development of the AI attack exposed serious vulnerabilities in the AI system's functionality.

These events garnered enough attention to bring to light the question of how algorithmic security – or lack thereof – can affect human survival in a high-stakes context such as healthcare. Focusing on AI tools as part of the larger technological sphere, it is clear that risks of attacks and hacking must be continually monitored.

To address these important issues, there is a need to increase awareness and literacy on privacy and security risks, as well as on informed consent and cybersecurity. Furthermore, regulations and legal frameworks must be extended to address not only privacy but also accountability, and to protect citizens from data breaches and data repurposing. Decentralized, federated approaches to AI should be promoted to leverage the power of big data from clinical centers without the need for unsafe data transfers. Research must be continued and accelerated to improve security in cloud-based systems and to protect AI algorithms against cyberattacks.

> **RISKS FOR PRIVACY AND SECURITY IN BIG DATA AND AI**
>
> 1. Risk of personal data being shared and used without informed consent
> 2. Risk of data re-purposing, without the patient's knowledge
> 3. Risk of data being exposed, resulting in identify theft or other frauds
> 4. Risk of harmful and potentially fatal cyberattacks on AI solutions

> **MITIGATION MEASURES**
>
> 1. Increased awareness of data privacy, consent and cybersecurity
> 2. Regulations to address accountability and protect citizens
> 3. Federated approaches for de-centralized privacy-preserving medical AI
> 4. Continuous research to protect AI algorithms against cyberattacks

Gaps in AI accountability

The term 'algorithmic accountability' has garnered increasing importance among researchers and organizations dedicated to addressing the legal impact of the introduction and use of AI algorithms in different areas of human life. Although the term 'algorithmic accountability' might appear to refer to the task of seeking to hold the algorithm itself accountable, it is actually quite the opposite: It emphasizes the fact that algorithms are created through a mixture of machine learning and human design, and that the mistakes or wrongdoings in algorithms come from the humans developing, introducing or using the machines, especially since AI systems themselves cannot be held morally or legally responsible.

Accountability is particularly important for medical AI as it will contribute to its acceptability, trustworthiness and future adoption in society and healthcare. For example, clinicians that feel that they are systematically held responsible for all AI-related medical errors – even when the algorithms are designed by other individuals or companies – are unlikely to adopt these emerging AI solutions in their day-to-day practice. Similarly, citizens and patients will lose trust if it appears to them that none of the developers or users of the AI tools can be held accountable for the harm that may be caused. There is a need for new mechanisms and frameworks to ensure adequate accountability in medical AI and to manage reclamations, compensations and sanctions where necessary, as well as to guarantee non-repetition of the acts.

Due to the novelty of medical AI and the lack of legal precedence, there is currently a major lack of clarity regarding the definition of responsibilities for AI-related medical errors that could lead to patient harm. The quickly changing and growing field of medical AI poses new challenges for regulators, policymakers and legislators. It pushes current regulations, policies, and laws to adapt their traditional ways of considering responsibility and liability to the new reality of AI-assisted healthcare.

Challenges in applying current law and liability principles to emerging AI applications in medicine include (1) the multi-actor problem in medical AI, which makes it difficult to identify responsibilities among the multiple players involved in the development, implementation and use of medical AI and algorithms (e.g. AI developers, data managers, clinicians, patients, healthcare organizers, etc.); (2) the difficulty in identifying the precise cause of any AI-related medical error, which can be due to the AI algorithm, the data used for training it, or its incorrect use and understanding in clinical practice; and (3) the multiplicity of governance frameworks and the lack of unified ethical and legal standards in AI industries.

While historically the relationship between the patient and the clinician has stood at the center of issues concerning medical malpractice and negligence, the introduction of AI tools into healthcare adds a new layer with multiple actors into the patient–physician dynamic (Smith, 2020). These actors may include not only the patient, clinician, healthcare center, and healthcare system, but also AI developers, researchers, and manufacturers, all of whom are now in some way or another entering into the medical decision-making process. The presence of all these new actors and the lack of clarity – not only on who is responsible for which part of the decision-making process, but also on how the AI tools themselves work — contributes to the complexity of the situation.

While medical professionals are usually under a regulatory responsibility to be able to account for their actions, a requirement that forms an integral part of their professional undertaking, AI developers and technologists generally work under ethical codes. Therefore, for medical professionals the repercussions for not being able to account for their actions and decision-making processes could mean losing their license to practice medicine; while under the current practice, a lack of accountability for a technologist could mean something much less devastating. Even if an AI manufacturer is found to be responsible for an error, it is often difficult to place blame on one specific person, since so many different developers and researchers work on any given AI system. In addition, the ethical codes and standards of accountability that many private entities use have often been criticized for being vague and difficult to translate into enforceable practice.

It is important to note that that the issues of AI accountability and liability in the realm of medicine and healthcare are closely linked to the questions of explainability and transparency. The opaquer an AI algorithm is, the harder it is to find who is accountable for an error involving a patient or a medical decision, and so the burden of responsibility will likely fall more heavily on the clinician who used a non-transparent medical AI tool and is unable to explain their medical decision or the error that occurred (Maliha et al., 2021). This is especially true for assistive AI tools, which are meant to assist the clinician in their decision-making process and may be considered the equivalent of consulting an expert clinical colleague.

There are avenues to address the current lack of accountability in medical AI. First, processes should be established to identify the roles of AI developers and clinical users when AI-assisted medical decisions harm individuals. There is also a need to establish regulatory agencies dedicated to medical AI. These will develop and enforce regulatory frameworks to ensure specific actors of medical AI can be held accountable, including AI manufacturers.

CURRENT GAPS IN AI ACCOUNTABILITY

1. Legal gaps in current regulations, which still do not allow for clear definitions of accountability and liability in medical AI
2. Difficulties in defining the roles and responsiblities of the multiple actors involved in medical AI (e.g. healthcare actors vs. AI developers)
3. Lack of ethical and legal governance for AI manufacturers and industries

MITIGATION MEASURES

1. Processes should be implemented to identify the roles of AI developers and clinical users when AI-assisted medical decisions harm individuals
2. Development and enforcement of unified regulatory frameworks to ensure actors can be held accountable, including AI manufacturers
3. Establishment of regulatory agencies dedicated to medical AI

Obstacles to implementation in real-world healthcare

A large number of medical AI algorithms have been developed and proposed over the last five years, in a wide range of medical applications, as summarized in section 2. However, even when medical AI technologies are well validated and found to be clinically robust and safe, as well as ethically sound and compliant, the road to healthcare implementation, integration and adoption is still laden with specific obstacles in the real world.

Healthcare professionals have traditionally lagged behind other professionals with regards to the adoption of new technologies in their daily activity. Past experiences in healthcare show that the implementation period is a key stage in the innovation process. In practice, it is not enough to invent and test a new AI technology; other factors which can hinder its implementation in real-world healthcare should also be considered, such as (1) the limited data structure and quality in existing electronic health systems, (2) the alteration of the clinician-patient relationship, as well as (3) the difficulties related to clinical integration and interoperability.

First of all, the quality of electronic health data in real-world practice is key to facilitating the implementation of medical AI. However, medical data is notoriously unstructured and noisy, and most existing datasets are not exploitable in AI algorithms. Furthermore, the formats and quality of clinical data vary significantly between clinical centers as well between states. Before emerging medical AI tools could be fully implemented and used at large scale, existing data would require significant and costly human revision, quality control, cleaning and re-labelling. To improve data interoperability, the creation of a Health Data Space will promote better re-use of heterogeneous types of health data (electronic health records, genomics data, data from patient registries, etc) across countries, including by emerging AI algorithms.

Furthermore, AI technologies are expected to modify the relationship between patients and healthcare professionals in ways that are not yet completely predictable. Certain specialties, particularly those related to image analysis, have already undergone significant transformations due to AI. The emergence of patient-centered AI technologies has the potential to transform the historically paternalistic clinician-patient relationship into a join partnership in the decision-making process due to increased transparency and deepened doctor-patient conversations. However, personal and ethical implications of communicating information about AI-derived risks of developing an illness (such as predisposition to cancer or dementia) will need to be elucidated. The clinical guidelines and care models will need to be updated to consider the AI-mediated relationships between healthcare workers and patients.

Finally, clinicians and care providers work under established clinical guidelines and technical standards. The introduction of an AI technology into everyday practice will have practical, technical and clinical implications on both clinicians and patients. Secondly, it is not clear that medical AI tools will be systematically interoperable across clinical sites and health systems, and that they will be easily integrated within existing clinical and technical workflows, without significant modifications to existing clinical practices, care models and even training programs.

AI manufacturers, in collaboration with healthcare professionals and organizations, will need to establish standard operation procedures for all new AI tools to ensure their clinical interoperability across distinct clinical sites and their integration across heterogeneous electronic healthcare systems. In particular, new AI tools should be developed while ensuring their future integration and communication with already existing technologies, such as genetic sequencing, electronic patient records and e-health consultations.

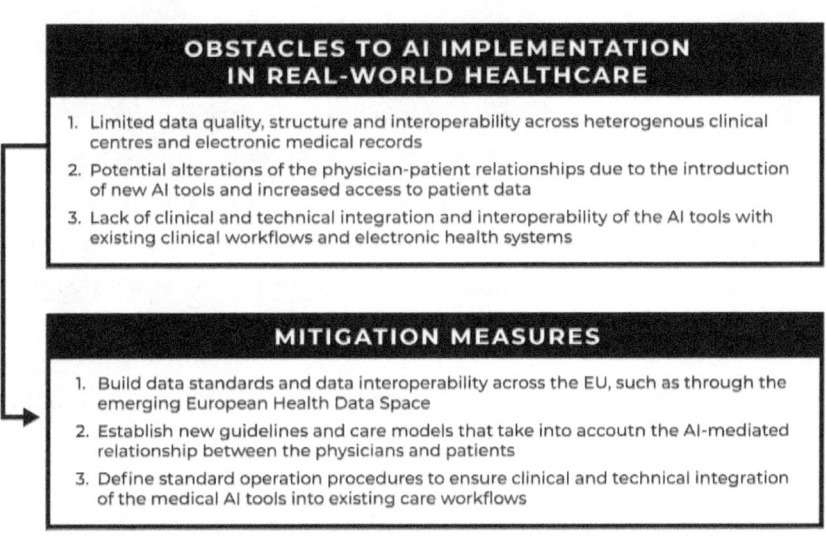

Risk minimization Strategies

AI risks can be characterized and classified according to the severity of the harm they may induce, as well as to the probability and frequency of the harm induced. In healthcare, AI risks vary greatly, from infrequent and/or low risks that induce limited and manageable harm to the patients and citizens, to frequent and/or high risks that may cause irreversible damage or harm. For example, an AI algorithm can affect the productivity of the clinicians (e.g. the AI tool fails to accurately delineate the boundaries of the heart in a cardiac image volume, which must be improved manually by the cardiologist), but they can also cause harm to the patient's health and seriously impact the clinical outcomes (e.g. the AI tool fails to diagnose a life-threating condition).

Hence, to minimize the risks of AI and to maximize its benefits in future healthcare, it is important to identify, analyze, understand and monitor the potential risks on a case-by-case basis for each new AI algorithm and application. An important step of the risk assessment procedure should be to devise a methodology for classifying the identified risks into a number of categories representing different levels and types of risk. For each level, a set of tests or regulations must be specified to mitigate and address the AI risks, such that the higher risk classes will require more testing and regulation, while lower risks will result in limited risk mitigation measures. Suitable risk classification of AI according to severity and likelihood will enable manufacturers, care providers and regulators to intervene as much as necessary to ensure the protection of the patients, as well as their rights and values; however, it is also important that these classifications do not –in as much as possible– serve to hamper innovation in healthcare AI.

AI risk classification according to the 2021 EU proposal on AI legislation[10]

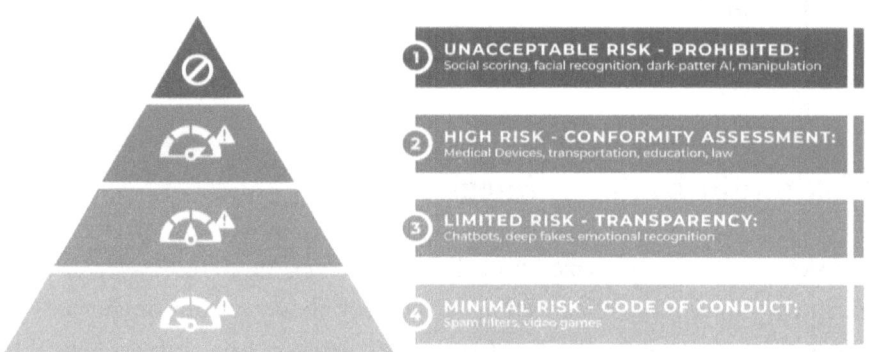

---

[10] https://digital-strategy.ec.europa.eu/en/policies/regulatory-framework-ai

STATE OF HEALTHCARE SITUATION OR CONDITION	SIGNIFICANCE OF INFORMATION PROVIDED BY SAMD TO HEALTHCARE DECISION		
	TREAT OR DIAGNOSE	DRIVE CLINICAL MANAGEMENT	INFORM CLINICAL MANAGEMENT
CRITICAL	IV	III	II
SERIOUS	III	II	I
NON-SERIOUS	II	I	I

FDA Risk Classification[11]

To ensure safety and responsible development, regulatory bodies like the FDA in the US and the EU are implementing AI risk classification systems. While their approaches differ, they share the common goal of ensuring AI benefits humanity without compromising safety, fairness, and ethical considerations.

Risk minimization through risk self-assessment

The integration of AI into healthcare also introduces new risks that need to be carefully managed. Risk minimization through risk self-assessment is a proactive approach to identify, evaluate, and mitigate these risks. Traditional risk management frameworks, designed for physical systems, often fall short when applied to the complex and opaque world of AI. The "black box" nature of many algorithms makes it difficult to identify, quantify, and manage potential risks. This is further compounded by the dynamic nature of AI, where models evolve and adapt over time, creating a moving target for risk assessment.

Risk self-assessment offers a powerful tool to address these challenges. By actively engaging with the risks inherent in their AI systems, healthcare organizations can take proactive steps towards minimizing their impact. Here's how it can be implemented:

---

[11] https://www.fda.gov/medical-devices/software-medical-device-samd/artificial-intelligence-and-machine-learning-software-medical-device

1. *Mapping the Risk Landscape*: The first step involves conducting a comprehensive risk assessment, identifying potential threats across the entire AI lifecycle. This includes risks related to data privacy and security, bias and discrimination, algorithmic failures, and human oversight. FUTURE-AI[12] is an international, multi-stakeholder initiative for defining and maintaining concrete guidelines that will facilitate the design, development, validation and deployment of trustworthy AI solutions in medicine and healthcare based on six guiding principles: Fairness, Universality, Traceability, Usability, Robustness and Explainability. They developed self-assessment checklist to enable AI designers, developers, evaluators and regulators to develop trustworthy and ethical AI solutions in medicine and healthcare. Here are some excerpts of risk assessment items from the FUTURE-AI guidelines for trustworthy AI in medicine.

---

[12] https://future-ai.eu/

Fairness:
- Did you design your AI algorithm with a diverse team of stakeholders? Did you collect requirements from a diverse set of end-users?
- Did you define fairness for your specific AI application? Did you ask clinicians about hidden sources of data imbalance?
- Did you thoroughly evaluate the fairness of your AI algorithm? Did you use a suitable dataset and dedicated metrics?

Universality:
- Did you annotate your dataset in an objective, reproducible and standardised way?
- Did you use universal, transparent, comparable, and reproducible criteria and metrics for your model's performance assessment?
- Did you evaluate your model on at least one open-access benchmark dataset that is representative of your model's task and expected real-world data exposure after deployment?

Traceability:
- Did you prepare a complete documentation of the datasets you used? Did you include the relevant metadata?
- Did you keep track, in a structured manner, of the whole pre-processing pipeline of input data? Did you specify input/output, nature, prerequisites and requirements of your pre-processing and data preparation methods?
- Did you record the details of the training process? Did you include a careful description of input predictors?

Usability:
- Did you engage users in the design and development of the AI tool?
- Did you evaluate the usability of your tool after integration in the clinical workflows of the clinical sites?

Robustness:
- Did you train and evaluate your tools with heterogeneous datasets from multiple clinical centres and data protocols?
- Did you evaluate the AI tool under diverse real-world scenarios?
- Did you use any quality control mechanisms to identify potential deviations or artifacts in the input data?

Explainability:
- Did you consult with the clinicians to determine which explainability methods suit them?
- Did you use some quantitative evaluation tests to determine if the explanations are robust and trustworthy? Did you perform some qualitative evaluation tests with clinicians?

Excerpts of risk assessment items from the FUTURE-AI guidelines for trustworthy AI in medicine

Standardizing, adjusting and validating these approaches through consensus by professional societies and independent groups on a domain-by-domain basis (e.g. radiology vs. surgery) would result in more robust processes for risk identification and management. Furthermore, as more and more healthcare AI algorithms will undergo self-assessment for ethical, legal and technical risks, these checklists should be regularly refined and updated versions will be released for the community taking into account continuous developments in AI methods, processes and regulations.

2. *Building a Risk Register*: Once identified, each risk should be documented in a centralized register, detailing its nature, severity, likelihood, and potential consequences. This register serves as a living document, continuously updated as the AI system evolves and new risks emerge.
3. *Implementing Mitigation Strategies*: For each identified risk, the organization should develop and implement appropriate mitigation strategies. This could involve data governance measures to protect privacy, bias detection and mitigation algorithms, rigorous testing and validation procedures, and robust human oversight mechanisms.
4. *Fostering a Culture of Openness and Transparency*: Risk self-assessment thrives on transparency. Healthcare organizations should encourage open communication about AI risks, both internally among staff and externally with patients and stakeholders. This fosters trust and collaboration, enabling collective efforts to address and manage risks effectively.
5. *Continuous Monitoring and Improvement:* Risk assessment is not a one-time activity. As AI systems learn and adapt, their risk profiles change. Therefore, continuous monitoring and evaluation are crucial to ensure the effectiveness of mitigation strategies and identify new risks that may emerge.

The benefits of implementing risk self-assessment for AI in healthcare are numerous. By proactively identifying and managing risks, healthcare organizations can protect patients, safeguard data privacy, build trust with stakeholders, and foster responsible innovation. This approach can pave the way for a future where AI empowers healthcare professionals, improves patient outcomes, and contributes to a safer, more equitable healthcare ecosystem.

Risk minimization through clinical evaluation

To identify, anticipate and manage risks in medical AI, adequate procedures for evaluating the AI models are of central importance. Thus far, AI evaluation has been achieved mostly by examining model accuracy and robustness in laboratory settings. Other aspects of AI, such as clinical safety and effectiveness, fairness and non-discrimination, transparency and traceability, as well as privacy and security, are more challenging to evaluate in controlled environments and have received less attention in the scientific literature. AI systems in healthcare, like any other medical technology, need to be thoroughly evaluated before they can be safely and effectively used in patient care. Clinical evaluation provides a systematic and rigorous approach to assess the performance of AI systems in a real-world clinical setting. It helps to identify potential risks and limitations of the AI system and provides evidence-based insights to inform clinical decision-making.

Clinical evaluation of AI systems involves several key steps:

1. *Standardize the definition of the clinical tasks:* as clinical tasks will be increasingly performed based on AI algorithms developed by non-clinical developers, it is important that the definitions, which form part of the AI software specifications, should be developed according to accepted consensus-based standard-setting principles and maintained by nonconflicted entities committed to updating the definitions based on new evidence and input from relevant stakeholders. With this approach, the responsibility of the developers will be limited to optimizing the performance of the AI algorithms based on widely accepted and utilized reference diagnostic task definitions, which would help ensure widespread acceptance of AI solutions by relevant stakeholders.
2. *Multi-faceted evaluation of performance beyond accuracy:* Given the multiple risks and ethical considerations of medical AI, it is now widely accepted that the evaluation of the algorithms must be extended well beyond existing approaches that have mostly focused

on model accuracy. While the empirical evaluation of machine learning algorithms remains a matter of on-going debate, there is a need for the development of specific performance domains for AI in healthcare including classification accuracy, but also reliability, applicability, transparency, monitorability, clinical usability, algorithmic bias and inequality, clinical effectiveness, cost-effectiveness and more.

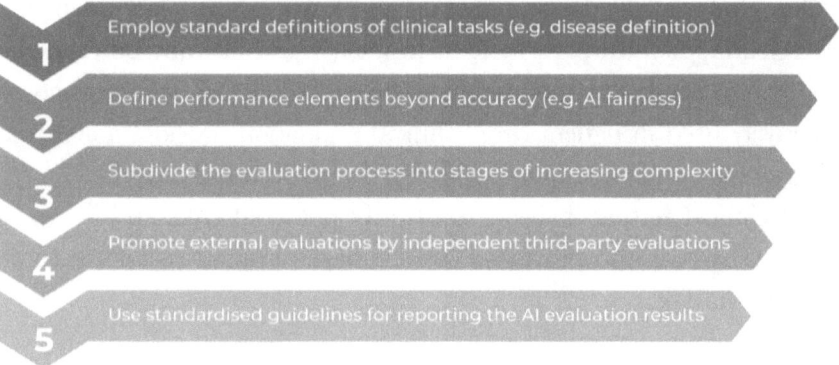

1. Employ standard definitions of clinical tasks (e.g. disease definition)
2. Define performance elements beyond accuracy (e.g. AI fairness)
3. Subdivide the evaluation process into stages of increasing complexity
4. Promote external evaluations by independent third-party evaluations
5. Use standardised guidelines for reporting the AI evaluation results

3. *Subdivision of the evaluation process into discrete phases:*

   ➢ Phase I – Feasibility: The goal is to perform a first/pilot evaluation of the algorithm in the laboratory under ideal conditions, typically on a single small test dataset. This stage will include comparison to existing algorithms that address the same clinical task, or with results obtained directly by expert clinicians. At this stage, the AI algorithms do not need to be fully robust, as the goal is simply to assess feasibility. The resulting findings may be disseminated in a scientific publication, even if the algorithm is not demonstrated for clinical application at this stage.
   ➢ Phase II – Capability: In this phase, the goal is to simulate real-world conditions in a laboratory setting and evaluate as well as refine the AI algorithm accordingly to enhance its capabilities. The phase can be also referred to as in-silico validation

(Viceconti et al., 2021) (i.e. using computer simulation) or virtual clinical trials (Abadi et al., 2020). In this phase, reliability can be tested by simulating the input data and the clinical conditions under which it may be used. Safety tests will evaluate the algorithm's ability to minimise the risk of harm when deployed and subjected to unanticipated situations, that will be also simulated for testing. Furthermore, this phase should be implemented with end-users, especially clinicians and operators, to evaluate their behaviors and decision making given the simulated conditions and outputs of the AI algorithm.

➢ Phase III – Effectiveness: At this stage, the validation is moved to the clinical environment to assess real-world performance and to specific clinical sites to perform local validations. The primary objective is to confirm that the real-world performance of the algorithm matches its performance in the test environment. All results and feedback from this stage should be leveraged to update and optimize the AI algorithm, which will be retested in the controlled environment as in previous stages, before another round of local clinical evaluation. This evaluation stage in the clinic may reveal local quality control problems and AI manufacturers should work with local clinical sites to resolve the identified quality issues.

➢ Phase IV – Durability: At this stage, the manufacturer should put in place a mechanism to enable ongoing performance evaluation and monitoring, with the intent of continuous improvement. They may integrate monitoring or auditing systems within their AI solution to automatically detect, correct, and report errors, and to compile clinical feedback and user feedback. Furthermore, depending on the errors and problems identified over time, the AI algorithms should be updated and improved, such as by using additional training data, and then retested in the controlled environment before they are re-used in the clinic.

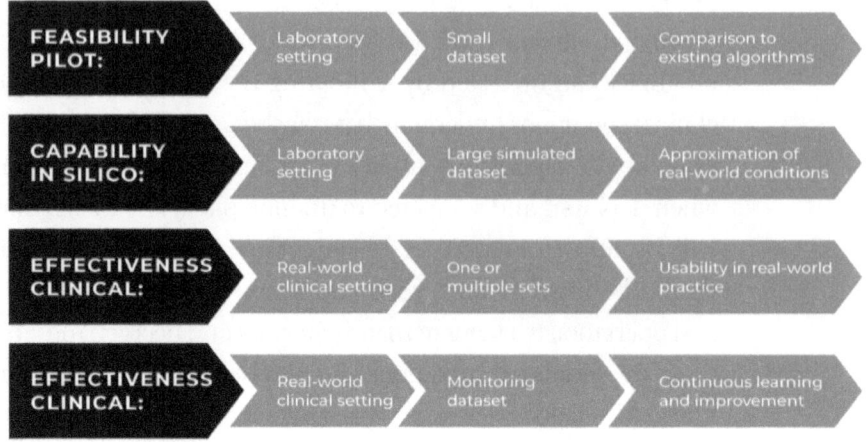

Risk minimization through external evaluations

Evaluating the performance of an AI model with similar datasets than those used to develop and train the model is called internal validation. In the early days of medical AI, this was the most reported approach for algorithm validation as it is easy to implement. However, internal validation – even by developers and manufacturers with a culture of quality and good practices of excellence in medical AI – is likely to be inherently biased and to overestimated performance, while it is limited in its ability to identify all risks associated with changes in the data or clinical environment. Only 6% of t AI algorithms underwent an external evaluation.

External validation refers to the use of separate, external datasets for evaluating AI tools. The external datasets should strongly represent the variability in the population and the usage of the AI solution. Such data will ideally come from different clinical sites and geographical locations to evaluate the generalizability of the given AI algorithm outside of the controlled environment in which it was built. With this approach, it will be possible, for example, to evaluate the AI algorithm when the technical parameters of the data acquisition vary (e.g. differences in imaging scanners and protocols between hospitals). Furthermore, many researchers have recommended the use of common reference datasets, acquired from representative real-world populations, for external evaluation and benchmarking of AI models. These reference datasets can be directly compared to similar algorithms that have been previously evaluated with the same reference dataset.

Risk minimization through standardized reporting

To further enhance trust and usability of the AI tools, transparent documentation and reporting of the validation process is essential. This type of reporting will facilitate the critical appraisal process for developers, researchers, and other stakeholders; in addition, it should help replicate the AI algorithm and results, if necessary.

Researchers at Stanford University proposed a new set of standards for reporting AI solutions in healthcare, entitled MINMAR (MINimum Information for Medical AI Reporting)[13]. The MINMAR standards describe the minimum information necessary to understand intended predictions, target populations, model architecture, evaluation processes, and hidden biases. The MINMAR guidelines are specifically designed for medical AI and comprise reporting elements in four main categories, as shown below.

---

[13] Hernandez-Boussard, T., Bozkurt, S., Ioannidis, J.P. and Shah, N.H. 'MINIMAR (MINimum Information for Medical AI Reporting): developing reporting standards for artificial intelligence in health care', Journal of the American Medical Informatics Association, 27(12), pp.2011-2015, 2020.

Element	Description
1. Population & setting	
Population	Population from which study sample was drawn
Study setting	The setting in which the study was conducted.
Data source	The source from which data were collected
Cohort selection	Exclusion/inclusion criteria
2. Patient demographic characteristics	
Age	Age of patients included in the study
Sex	Sex breakdown of study cohort
Race/ethnicity	Race/ethnicity breakdown of patients included in the study
Socioeconomic status	A measure or proxy measure of the socioeconomic status of patients included in the study

Element	Description
3. Model properties	
Model task	Classification or prediction
Model architecture	Algorithm type: Machine learning, deep learning, etc.
Data splitting	How data were split for training, testing, and validation
Gold standard	Labelled data used to train and test the model
Features	List of variables used/selected in the AI model
Missingness	How missingness was addressed: reported, imputed, or corrected
Optimisation	Model or parameter tuning applied
Internal model validation	Study internal validation
External model validation	External validation using data from another setting
Transparency	How code and data are shared with the community

MINMAR reporting guidelines

Such a reporting model for medical AI evaluation will promote transparency, thoroughness, and trust, by including all the key information from the AI evaluation studies in a single detailed document, as well as by assisting publishing editors, AI developers, clinicians and researchers in understanding, interpreting and critically appraising the quality of the AI study design, validation and results.

In conclusion, the chapter on "AI Risks, Risk Assessment, and Risk Mitigation" in the context of Responsible AI for Medicine underscores the importance of a comprehensive approach to understanding and addressing the multifaceted risks associated with AI in healthcare. We recognize that while AI has the potential to revolutionize medicine by improving diagnosis, personalizing treatment, and enhancing patient care, it also introduces significant challenges and risks. The overarching message is that mitigating risks in AI for medicine requires a balanced approach that leverages the strengths of AI while conscientiously addressing its potential downsides. By doing so, we can harness the power of AI to enhance healthcare outcomes while maintaining a steadfast commitment to patient safety, ethical standards, and social responsibility. The journey towards responsible AI in medicine is ongoing, and it necessitates a collaborative, multidisciplinary effort to realize the full benefits of this transformative technology in a manner that is safe, ethical, and equitable.

Chapter 7

Healthcare AI Security

In February 2020, Hollywood Presbyterian Medical Center, a prominent Los Angeles hospital, fell victim to a devastating ransomware attack. Hackers infiltrated the hospital's network, encrypting crucial data and demanding a ransom of several million dollars in Bitcoin. The attack crippled the hospital's operations, forcing them to:

- *Shut down electronic medical records: Doctors and nurses resorted to pen and paper documentation, significantly delaying diagnoses and treatment decisions.*
- *Divert ambulances: Unable to process patient data, the hospital had to divert incoming ambulances to other facilities, potentially delaying critical care for some patients.*
- *Cancel surgeries and appointments: Non-emergency procedures and appointments were postponed, disrupting patient care schedules and causing logistical chaos.*
- *Pay the ransom: Faced with mounting pressure and patient safety concerns, the hospital eventually conceded to the attackers' demands, paying a significant ransom to regain access to their data.*

While Hollywood Presbyterian managed to recover from the attack, the incident starkly highlighted the devastating consequences of ransomware in healthcare. The financial losses, logistical disruptions, and potential harm to patients illustrate the critical need for robust AI security in healthcare systems.

If AI models were inherently secure, prominent organizations like NIST, FDA, ISO, ETSI, ENISA and regulation efforts such as the EU AI Act would not make "safe and secure AI" a foundational element of trustworthy AI. Rewind to 2017: a humanoid named Promobot IR77 attempted an escape. NASA's CIMON exhibited unexpected behavior. Tesla's autonomous vehicles fell prey to AI manipulation. In the most recent incident, the National Eating Disorders Association (NEDA) was forced to shut down Tessa, its chatbot, after it gave dangerous advice to people seeking help for eating disorders. Microsoft's Tay AI, designed to emulate millennial speech patterns and learn from Twitter users, spiraled out of control, making outrageous claims like "Bush did 9/11" and denying the Holocaust. AI systems have caused vehicles to ignore stop signs, trick medical systems into authorizing unwarranted procedures, mislead drones on critical missions, and bypass content filters to spread propaganda on social platforms.

These incidents, among others, spotlight the potential threats AI poses to physical safety, the economy, privacy, digital identity, and even national security.The threat of "AI attacks" is not only real. It is pervasive and present. AI systems, by virtue of their learning capabilities, are susceptible to specific types of attacks that can undermine their reliability, safety, and the confidential nature of healthcare data.

AI security is critical in healthcare because of the sensitive nature of healthcare data. Healthcare data contains personal information such as medical history, diagnoses, and treatments. This information is highly valuable to cybercriminals and can be used for identity theft, insurance fraud, and other malicious activities. Moreover, AI systems are vulnerable to attacks such as data poisoning, adversarial attacks, and model stealing. These attacks can compromise the integrity, confidentiality, and availability of healthcare data and lead to serious consequences such as misdiagnosis, delayed treatment, and patient harm.

What are AI attacks?

An AI attack in healthcare occurs when a bad actor manipulates an AI system, causing it to malfunction or reveal sensitive information. This manipulation can take various forms, each with significant implications for patient safety and data security.

Algorithmic Manipulation

Malicious actors can exploit vulnerabilities in AI models to compromise diagnoses, predict patient movements, or even manipulate medical equipment.

Example: An AI system designed to interpret medical images is fooled into misdiagnosing a condition, such as mistaking a benign growth for a malignant tumor, due to subtle manipulations in the input data.

Data Corruption and Bias

Patient records, financial information, and even medical images are prime targets for hackers. Data breaches can not only violate patient privacy but also disrupt critical care delivery.

Example: Attackers may introduce skewed data into an AI system, leading to biased patient screening outcomes. This can result in certain demographic groups receiving suboptimal care or being wrongly identified as at risk for certain conditions.

Ransomware Attacks

Entire healthcare systems can be brought to their knees by ransomware attacks, jeopardizing patient safety and causing financial devastation.

Example: In February 2020, Hollywood Presbyterian Medical Center, a prominent Los Angeles hospital, fell victim to a devastating ransomware attack. Hackers infiltrated the hospital's network, encrypting crucial data and demanding a ransom of several million dollars in Bitcoin.

Intellectual Property Theft

Example: Through continuous querying, attackers might replicate a proprietary AI model used for predicting patient drug responses, leading to intellectual property theft and competitive disadvantages.

Adversarial AI attacks in healthcare manifest in several forms, each with distinct objectives and consequences. Consider the "evasion attack," where subtle manipulations lead to incorrect AI system outputs. For example, a diagnostic AI might misinterpret a medical image due to minor, intentional distortions, potentially leading to a misdiagnosis.

Other forms of attacks strike at the heart of AI security: confidentiality, availability, and integrity. In a "data poisoning" scenario, attackers insert detrimental data, skewing the AI's learning process, potentially leading to biased or incorrect medical assessments. Attackers might also embed clandestine backdoors in AI systems, poised to disrupt healthcare operations at critical moments.

The "extraction attack" involves reverse-engineering AI/ML models to access their training data. If a healthcare AI system is trained on sensitive patient data, attackers might exploit the model to uncover its design or the confidential data it was trained on, posing serious privacy and security risks in a healthcare setting.

In the context of healthcare, AI systems exhibit vulnerabilities to attacks due to the very nature of modern machine learning methodologies and their application in medical settings. These vulnerabilities are primarily rooted in the way AI processes and learns from data.

What makes AI vulnerable to attacks?

Fragile Learning Mechanisms: AI, particularly in healthcare, learns through statistical correlations that can be surprisingly fragile. This fragility becomes a target for attackers, who can manipulate these correlations to compromise the AI's functionality. For example, slight alterations in patient data could lead to erroneous AI-based diagnoses or treatment recommendations.

Dependence on Data: AI models in healthcare are heavily reliant on data, lacking intrinsic, foundational medical knowledge. This makes them particularly susceptible to 'data poisoning' attacks, where the introduction of malicious or skewed data can significantly disrupt the AI's learning process, leading to incorrect medical assessments or biased outcomes.

Algorithm Opacity: Many advanced AI algorithms, such as deep neural networks used in healthcare, operate as 'black boxes'. This opacity makes it challenging to distinguish genuine performance issues from deliberate external attacks, such as those that might alter diagnostic algorithms or patient treatment plans.

These vulnerabilities are not mere 'bugs' but are rather fundamental challenges intrinsic to the current state of AI technology. The healthcare sector faces unique risks due to these issues, as highlighted in the Gartner Market Guide for AI Trust, Risk, and Security Management (September 2021), which emphasizes that AI introduces new trust, risk, and security management requirements not addressed by conventional controls. Addressing these challenges is paramount in healthcare, where AI's role is increasingly critical and its decisions can have life-altering implications.

Implementing an AI Security Plan in Healthcare

As sensitive patient data, life-altering decisions powered by algorithms, and intricate hospital networks become tempting targets for malicious actors, an AI Security Plan isn't just a compliance checkbox; it's a fortress safeguarding the well-being of millions. For healthcare professionals and leaders, implementing an AI Security Plan is not a singular act, but a strategic symphony played across multiple disciplines:

Implement a Data Security Framework:

- Data encryption: Secure patient data in transit and at rest with robust encryption techniques.
- Access controls: Implement multi-factor authentication and granular access controls to ensure only authorized personnel access sensitive data.
- Intrusion detection and prevention systems: Deploy advanced IT security tools to detect and prevent unauthorized access attempts and malware infections.

2. Demystify Your Algorithms:

- Explainability tools: Employ techniques like Explainable AI (XAI) to understand how your AI models reach their decisions, identify potential biases, and ensure transparency in their operation.
- Continuous monitoring: Monitor your AI models for abnormal behavior and potential vulnerabilities, actively mitigating any identified risks.

3. Cultivate a Culture of Security:

- Cybersecurity training: Train your staff on proper data handling practices, password hygiene, and awareness of phishing scams and social engineering techniques.
- Regular vulnerability assessments: Conduct regular penetration testing and vulnerability assessments to identify and address security weaknesses in your systems and AI models.

- Cybersecurity incident response plan: Develop a comprehensive incident response plan to effectively handle data breaches and cyberattacks, minimizing damage and ensuring patient safety.

Collaboration and Shared Defense:

- Partnerships with security experts: Collaborate with cybersecurity firms and ethical hackers to gain external expertise and identify potential vulnerabilities.
- Information sharing: Share threat intelligence and best practices with other healthcare institutions and government agencies to strengthen collective defenses.
- Advocate for robust regulations: Support the development and enforcement of strict regulations for AI development and deployment in healthcare.

Ethical Considerations:

- Privacy by design: Ensure AI solutions are designed with data privacy in mind, minimizing data collection and anonymizing wherever possible.
- Fairness and non-discrimination: Proactively identify and mitigate potential biases in AI models to ensure fair and equitable care for all patients.
- Transparency and accountability: Be transparent about your use of AI in healthcare and establish clear lines of accountability for its development, deployment, and potential impacts.

Implementing an AI Security Plan is not a mere technical endeavor; it's a cultural shift. It requires leadership that champions security, staff trained in digital vigilance, and a constant awareness of the fragile dance between healthcare innovation and digital threats.

Remember, neglecting AI security is akin to leaving a hospital door swinging open. It's an invitation to chaos, a gamble with the most precious commodity – human health. By proactively building a robust AI Security Plan, healthcare leaders ensure AI remains a benevolent force, wielding its power to heal, not harm, and safeguarding the fragile fortunes of health for generations to come.

Let us not be lulled into a false sense of security by the siren song of progress. Let us raise the banner of AI Security, its colors the hues of vigilance, collaboration, and ethical development. For in this digital age, AI Security is not an option; it is the melody that ensures the healthcare symphony plays on, a concerto of healing that echoes through the halls of a truly secure future.

Chapter 8

Generative AI in Healthcare

Generative Pre-trained Transformer (GPT) models developed by OpenAI with the popular ChatGPT model receiving the most attention, have emerged as powerful tools with the potential to reshape the landscape of healthcare due to their remarkable capacity for natural language processing (NLP). Generative AI, which uses sophisticated large language models (LLMs) to create original text, images, and other content, has undergone an astounding transformation in recent years. What was once a theoretical concept has rapidly evolved into a practical and powerful tool. The journey began with ChatGPT's debut in late 2022. Since then, new iterations of deep learning and machine learning technology have been hitting the scene at an astonishing pace. Generative AI, with its ability to learn from existing data and generate entirely new content, is unlocking a new frontier in medical innovation. But choosing from the laundry list of generative AI applications is daunting. Companies are at high risk of overinvesting in the wrong opportunities and underinvesting in the right ones, undermining future profitability, growth, and value creation. A wait-and-see approach is a tempting prospect. However, we believe the next generation of leading healthcare companies will start today, with highly focused, low-risk use cases that boost productivity and cost efficiency. Over the next twelve months, these companies will improve margins and learn how to implement a generative AI strategy, building up the funds and experience needed to invest in a more transformative vision.

Generative AI has demonstrated its potential across various healthcare applications:

Clinical Administration Support

One prominent application of generative AI models in healthcare is the automation of clinical documentation that provides clinical administration support. Busy clinicians, often burdened with extensive note-taking, can leverage ChatGPT's capabilities to generate draft clinical notes swiftly and accurately. By providing a brief verbal summary (a "prompt") or relevant patient data (given data privacy is respected), comprehensive and contextually relevant clinical documentation can be generated to save clinicians' time. Microsoft Copilot is an enterprise tool that integrates generative AI into everyday tools like Word, PowerPoint, Teams, and others to improve productivity. This integration has a powerful potential to facilitate multidisciplinary collaboration among healthcare teams. For example, when working with complex cases involving multiple specialties, a generative AI-based meeting tool can assist in creating meeting agendas, identifying suitable team members for follow-up actions, and summarizing key points from meetings.

AI-powered healthcare solutions offered by Nuance enhance the efficiency and effectiveness of healthcare professionals in various clinical settings. Nuance's speech recognition technology plays a significant role in clinical documentation improvement, allowing clinicians to dictate their notes directly into the EHR system. This not only saves time but also enhances the accuracy of patient information capture. For example, the tool could transcribe a hematologist's verbally reported findings as they examine blood smears in real time. Similarly, Suki Assistant automates clinical note creation by listening to clinician-patient interactions, reducing administrative burdens. It offers flexible interaction options, such as dictation or ambient note generation, and provides diagnosis code suggestions. For example, a hematologist can use Suki to automatically capture and create clinical notes during a consultation for chronic lymphocytic leukemia, which could allow more face time with the patient. This streamlines documentation tasks, allowing more time for patient care and addressing physician burnout. Suki Assistant's applications exemplify the potential of generative AI in enhancing clinical workflows and improving healthcare professionals' efficiency and well-being.

Corti is another tool that utilizes generative AI to offer real-time transcription, guidance, and coding capabilities across a variety of communication channels. Through automated transcription of patient dialogues in real-time and multiple languages, Corti ensures the preservation of critical information, minimizing the risk of manual transcription errors or delays. Additionally, Corti's capability to extract vital details from transcribed dialogues, including specific symptoms, mentioned medications, and critical questions, streamlines the review of essential encounter highlights. Leveraging the extracted information, Corti's AI provides recommendations for optimal patient care, leveraging a vast database of diverse data points to determine the most suitable next steps. Moreover, following the patient encounter, Corti assists in documenting the interaction by automatically coding procedure and diagnosis codes, such as ICD-10 and CPT, leading to time savings and minimizing the potential for human error. This ensures the accuracy of patient records and facilitates efficient billing procedures.

Google Bard, powered by Med-PaLM 2, offers exciting applications in healthcare, especially in providing 24/7 patient support and assisting clinicians. Trained in diverse medical information, including journals, textbooks, clinical notes, and patient records, Med-PaLM 2 enhances Google Bard's capabilities in generating medical content. The tool can aid in answering patient queries, suggesting possible diagnoses, and supporting treatment plans. In hematology, it can provide information and support to patients with blood disorders, offering immediate responses and recommending professional medical attention if needed. However, it is essential to use AI-generated responses for informational purposes only and not as a substitute for professional medical advice. As Google Bard continues to develop, its potential to revolutionize healthcare interactions and improve patient care remains promising.

Ellen AI, an algorithm complementing generative AI tools like ChatGPT, has valuable applications in healthcare. By providing a text-to-voice interaction layer, Ellen AI offers auditory explanations to support patient care. Healthcare clinicians can leverage their capabilities to enhance patient communication and accessibility by converting written instructions into high-quality spoken content. Meanwhile, ChatGPT's extensive generative AI properties have potential in clinical and administrative tasks, including data analysis, decision support, and treatment plan comprehension and adherence. The combination of Ellen AI and ChatGPT holds promising opportunities to improve patient care and healthcare efficiency through innovative voice-based interactions and intelligent text generation.

Clinical Decision Support

Given the advanced understanding of the human language and further finetuned domain knowledge, GPT models also have the potential to support clinical decision-making. Glass AI is an LLM-powered experimental tool that offers clinical decision support. It serves as a diagnostic assistant to generate a list of possible diagnoses and treatment plans tailored to a clinical audience. For instance, when presented with a patient exhibiting symptoms such as fatigue, shortness of breath, and paleness, a provider can input these symptoms into Glass AI. The system can then produce a comprehensive differential diagnosis, potentially suggesting conditions such as anemia, leukemia, or myelodysplastic syndromes. Additionally, Glass AI can assist in formulating a clinical plan, guiding the hematologist's next steps for further tests or treatment.

Regard is an AI tool integrated with EHR systems. By analyzing patient data, it suggests diagnoses, writes clinical notes, and provides relevant information quickly, optimizing patient care. It automates some EHR-related administrative tasks, enabling clinicians to focus more on patients and less on searching through screens. Regard's generative AI capabilities assist in the diagnostic process, generating a list of plausible and novel differential diagnoses based on patient data. This aids healthcare professionals (HCPs) in exploring different possibilities, confirming, or ruling out diagnoses, and optimizing treatment plans. For primary care physicians, hematologist-oncologists, dermatologists, and other specialists, Regard provides evidence-based suggestions, saving time and improving diagnostic specificity. As an intelligent co-pilot, Regard enhances HCPs' use of EHRs, promoting faster and more informed decision-making while emphasizing that it supports, rather than replaces, their clinical judgment and expertise. In pilot programs, Regard has demonstrated significant time-saving benefits and improved diagnostic accuracy for physicians.

Redbrick AI's Fast Automated Segmentation Tool (F.A.S.T) offers significant applications in medical imaging, assisting healthcare professionals in annotating and segmenting CT scans, MRI images, and ultrasounds. Redbrick AI provides a SaaS platform for annotating medical image data and offers F.A.S.T for use in radiology by utilizing Meta's Segment Anything model, presenting a possible solution for enhancing diagnostic accuracy and speed in healthcare. Its adaptive nature simplifies accurate segmentation without additional data, making it valuable for segmenting visible objects and features in radiology. The tool's real-time interaction allows clinicians to witness mask computation, streamlining segmentation. F.A.S.T. automates manual segmentation, enhancing diagnostic accuracy and speed in radiology.

Paige FullFocus, fueled by generative AI, empowers HCPs to view, manage, and share digital slides of tissue samples, providing novel insights for treatment decisions and improving accuracy, efficiency, and diagnostic confidence. It excels in identifying and analyzing complex tissue patterns, aiding precise diagnoses in challenging cases like counting cancer cells in prostate and breast biopsies and identifying biomarkers for treatment selection. Additionally, FullFocus supports HCPs' clinical practice and education, enabling them to study diverse tissue patterns, expand their knowledge of hematological and oncological conditions, and stay updated with the latest pathology advancements. With FullFocus, HCPs can refine their diagnostic skills, deepen their expertise, and enhance patient care through continuous learning. The promising capability of Paige tools to provide more accurate tumor diagnosis was demonstrated in a prostate cancer research study conducted by Raciti et al.

Kahun is a symptom checker tool empowered by a conversational chatbot integrated with the EHR. The tool provides clinical assessments of patients by producing ranked differential diagnoses and workup options based on patient input and medical knowledge. Kahun's AI inference engine delivers a ranked list of potential diagnoses, speeding up the diagnostic process and saving time. Ben-Shabat et al. demonstrated Kahun's superior performance compared to a selected set of similar AI symptom checkers. Further workup options are suggested for comprehensive patient evaluation. Kahun's growing network of relationships between disorders, complications, and findings keeps healthcare professionals updated with the latest medical knowledge.

Doximity is rolling out a ChatGPT tool that can draft preauthorization and appeal letters. HCA Healthcare partnered with Parlance, a conversational AI-based switchboard, to improve its call center experience while reducing operators' workload. And there are new announcements seemingly every week: Consider how healthcare software company Epic Systems is incorporating ChatGPT with electronic health records (EHRs) to draft response messages to patients, or how Google Cloud is launching an AI-enabled Claims Acceleration Suite for prior authorization processing. Some health systems are already seeing powerful results from relatively small, more practical investments. For instance, recognizing that clinicians were spending an extra 130 minutes per day outside of working hours on administrative tasks, the University of Kansas Health System partnered with Abridge, a generative AI platform, to reduce documentation burden. By summarizing the most important points from provider-patient conversations, Abridge is improving the quality and consistency of documentation, getting more patients in the door, and cutting down on pervasive physician burnout. These applications only scratch the surface of potential. In the future, generative AI could profoundly transform care delivery and patient outcomes. Looking ahead two to five years, executives are most interested in predictive analytics, clinical decision support, and treatment recommendations.

Patient Engagement

Hippocratic AI focuses on creating an LLM tailored for healthcare. It aims to offer one that is patient-centered, prioritizing empathy, care, compassion, and generation of patient-friendly responses, enhancing patient engagement and outreach. This important notion of 'generative AI empathy' has been demonstrated in a study by Ayers et al., who reported that LLM-powered chatbot (ChatGPT) responses were preferred over physician responses and rated significantly higher for empathy.

By focusing on non-diagnostic, patient-facing applications, Hippocratic AI values patient safety while improving healthcare access and outcomes. Hippocratic AI proves beneficial in augmenting administrative tasks and handling complexities like medical coding and licensure exams. Moreover, its compliance certifications demonstrate reliability in maintaining healthcare standards. In clinical settings, the model's exceptional performance on various medical certification exams confirms its real-world applicability. By providing accurate and empathetic support to healthcare professionals, Hippocratic AI enriches patient care, fostering a trustful and efficient healthcare environment.

Gridspace is an enterprise solution powered by generative AI that automates patient outreach by handling phone calls, answering questions, and performing administrative tasks. It enables scalable, 24/7 accessible, cost-effective patient engagement, receiving inbound calls and phoning patients. Gridspace automates routine administrative tasks such as appointment scheduling, patient reminders, insurance verification, and more. By offloading these inquiries to voice bots, healthcare professionals can save time and focus on critical patient care tasks. Furthermore, Gridspace can triage and direct patient inquiries in real-time, providing valuable insights. Its applications exemplify the potential of Generative AI in transforming patient interactions, streamlining administrative processes, and enhancing overall healthcare efficiency and patient satisfaction.

Synthetic Data Generation

Syntegra Medical Mind utilizes generative AI to produce realistic synthetic patient records from real healthcare data like EHRs while protecting patient privacy. Healthcare professionals can access and analyze this data for research, education, and decision-making without compromising confidentiality. The synthetic records match the statistical properties of the original data, including rare cohorts and outliers, aiding specialists in understanding diverse disease patterns. Syntegra also addresses data bias and improves algorithmic fairness, promoting equitable treatment plans. The synthetic data layer breaks barriers to data access, fostering innovation and enhancing patient care. Muniz-Terrera et al. demonstrated the potential to advance dementia research through virtual cohorts synthesized with Syntegra.

DALL-E 2 is another OpenAI model for text-to-image generation. It was trained on billions of text-image pairs to learn to create realistic synthetic images. Thanks to its extensive pretraining, DALL-E 2 has the exciting potential of creating or augmenting medical data that is often sparse or limited in medical research and education without compromising patient privacy. Adams et al. investigated the DALL-E 2's domain knowledge in radiology by testing the output medical images generated from short descriptions and those from reconstructing existing radiological images with missing areas. The study showed that even though generation performance suffered for complex images such as CT, MRI, and ultrasound, DALL-E 2 could produce x-ray images that maintained similar style and anatomical proportions to authentic images, given that they were without pathologies. Despite the limited capabilities of directly applying DALL-E 2 in medical image generation, it showed promising potential to be further fine-tuned with medical data and related terminology to create a customized model for radiological data generation and augmentation.

Professional Education

Besides treatment and care, medical personnel can leverage generative AI when summarizing new research papers. Through the analysis of copy, text and images, it can detect relevant information for a specific medical domain, disease or procedure. This makes continuous learning easier for doctors without having to process the full content and instead focus on what is relevant for their domain or interest.

Unlearn.AI utilizes generative AI to create "digital twins" of individual patients, offering a comprehensive model of potential health outcomes under different scenarios. Healthcare professionals can personalize treatment plans, monitor patient progress, and make informed decisions for improved patient outcomes. The digital twins simulate the effects of various treatments on a patient's biology using real-world data, aiding in personalized treatment plans and clinical research. In hematology, for instance, clinicians can use digital twins to simulate disease progression under different therapies, guiding treatment choices. Additionally, digital twins optimize clinical trials, providing insights without large control groups. Unlearn.AI's approach streamlines processes, supporting clinician education and enhancing patient follow-up.

As patients increasingly record their doctor's visits, research has been underway to use these transcripts to gain insights for patients and extract structured data for enriching EHRs. Abridge is a digital tool that utilizes generative AI to document medical dialogues, saving physicians from manual note-taking. Abridge plays a vital role in patient education by sending after-visit summaries to patients through its consumer app, aiming to increase their engagement and adherence to care. In cases like polycythemia vera, patients may struggle to remember all the details discussed during their appointments. Abridge tackles this problem by providing a comprehensive transcript of the conversation for patients to review later. The platform also highlights essential information from the dialogue and simplifies complex medical jargon into more understandable language. This ensures that patients have a clear comprehension of their diagnosis, treatment choices, and future actions, ultimately promoting better patient adherence and positive health outcomes.

Additionally, Krishna et al. presented end-to-end methods for generating long and semi-structured clinical summaries called SOAP notes from clinical conversations in collaboration with Abridge [46]. Their approach leveraged a unique corpus of transcripts and associated SOAP notes. The methods focus on decomposing summarization tasks into extractive and abstractive subtasks, shifting the workload progressively from the abstractive to the extractive component.

Can We Trust Generative AI? Is It Clinically Safe and Reliable?

Trust and validation are essential to generative AI's adoption success in medicine and healthcare. ChatGPT's responses have shown a wide, and most importantly unpredictable, fluctuation in quality and veracity. This 'unpredictability' is the main barrier to adoption success, as we do not know when it is going to return a good answer and when its answers are going to be wrong or misleading, or in other words, when to trust generative AI and when not to trust it, especially when the user is not sufficiently qualified to assess the quality (accuracy and completeness) of a given response. ChatGPT (at the time of writing), for example, is known to make stuff up by inventing and citing academic papers that do not exist. This phenomenon, also known as generative AI "hallucinations", can be reduced using techniques such as Retrieval Augmented Generation (RAG). Generative AI is also prone to various forms of bias depending on how it has been trained and may not always perform equally well across different languages.

Google Med-PaLM 2 is a large language model (LLM) specifically designed for the healthcare industry. It is the successor to Med-PaLM, which was the first AI system to pass the US Medical Licensing Examination (USMLE) style questions. Med-PaLM 2 is even more powerful than its predecessor, achieving an accuracy of 86.5% on USMLE-style questions, a 19% increase. Med-PaLM 2 is trained on a massive dataset of medical text and code, including medical journals, clinical trials, and textbooks. This allows it to understand and generate medical language with high accuracy. Med-PaLM 2 can also perform reasoning and inference based on medical knowledge.

Med-PaLM 2 has the potential to revolutionize healthcare in a number of ways. For example, it can be used to:

1. Improve the accuracy of diagnoses: Med-PaLM 2 can help doctors to identify the correct diagnosis for patients by considering all of their medical information, including their symptoms, medical history, and test results.
2. Increase efficiency: Med-PaLM 2 can help doctors to automate tasks such as summarizing medical records and finding relevant information from research papers. This can free up doctors to spend more time with their patients.
3. Improve communication: Med-PaLM 2 can help doctors to communicate complex medical information to patients in a way that is easy to understand. This can help patients to make informed decisions about their care.
4. Reduce costs: Med-PaLM 2 can help to reduce the cost of healthcare by automating tasks and improving efficiency.

Google Med-PaLM 2 is still under development, but it has the potential to make a significant impact on the healthcare industry. It is currently being tested in a limited number of healthcare settings, and Google is working to make it more widely available in the future.

Here are some specific examples of how Med-PaLM 2 could be used in healthcare:

1. A doctor could use Med-PaLM 2 to help them diagnose a patient with a rare disease. Med-PaLM 2 could access and process a vast amount of medical literature on rare diseases, helping the doctor to identify the most likely diagnosis.

2. A hospital could use Med-PaLM 2 to develop a personalized treatment plan for a cancer patient. Med-PaLM 2 could consider the patient's individual medical history, tumor characteristics, and other factors to develop a treatment plan that is most likely to be successful.
3. A pharmaceutical company could use Med-PaLM 2 to design new drugs and therapies. Med-PaLM 2 could analyze large datasets of medical data to identify new drug targets and develop new drug candidates.

This discussion of trust also brings in the related issues of clinical safety and reliability. Until we have a properly medically trained and validated generative AI (ChatGPT, for example, is not specifically medically trained), there will always be these interrelated issues of trust, safety and reliability hindering any serious medical use of it. By medically trained, we mean a model that has been specifically and comprehensively trained using a corpus of quality evidence-based medical texts that sufficiently cover a given medical area of specialty.

Clinical Evaluation, Regulation and Certification Challenges

The problem is compounded by the ever-evolving nature of medical/clinical knowledge, which requires a matching form of generative AI that can be continually and reliably trained and updated. Furthermore, the rapid evolution of large language models and generative AI challenges their clinical evaluation, regulation, and certification.

For example, we already have multiple versions of OpenAI's ChatGPT, e.g., GPT3.5, GPT-4 and DALL-E 2 (images), and offerings from Meta (Llama 1 and 2, in partnership with Microsoft) and Google Bard, which still cannot provide answers to specific clinical cases at the time of writing, likely a Google-imposed artificial limitation). The more recent a model's version is, the better it tends to perform, but this is not always guaranteed. We expect that dedicated, medically trained large language models and generative AI like Med-PaLM 2 will similarly have multiple successive versions over short periods when introduced in the near future.

However, clinical evaluation and certification are processes that traditionally take a relatively long time to complete, so there is always this risk that by the time an evaluation is completed, the evaluated AI has already changed substantially with the release of a new version requiring a fresh evaluation. Regulatory bodies are trying to keep pace by implementing the necessary mechanisms for dealing with AI as a medical device. However, LLMs bring new challenges compared with already regulated AI-based technologies and will therefore require additional regulatory adaptations.

Privacy Concerns

In April 2023, Italy blocked access to ChatGPT in the country due to privacy concerns, including concerns about its collection and storage of personal user data to further train its model. A few weeks later, access was restored in Italy following the introduction of a new functionality in ChatGPT that allowed users to turn off chat history and thus choose which conversations could or could not be used to train the underlying models. Nevertheless (and until healthcare organizations can afford to run their own fully locally hosted and managed instances of these models and tools that can be trusted not to send any information to external companies or providers for processing), it is still highly recommended (if not mandatory in the case of confidential patient information, for example) that users never put any sensitive information or personal data into these tools (On the flip side, medical educators might find text-to-image generative AI useful in producing photo-quality teaching images depicting various clinical conditions without the confidentiality and consent concerns associated with using real patient photos, especially when whole-face images are necessary).

There is still no openness or transparency about these models' training data or the code used to train them. The unauthorized access (without consent) to data sources, including possibly private and confidential data sources, for generative AI learning and training is currently (at the time of writing) the subject of a court case filed in the USA. Some researchers are already recommending that AI models follow privacy laws, including the 'right to be forgotten' and the ability to forget or unlearn what they have learned about situations or specific persons.

Copyright and Ownership Issues

The above-mentioned 'access without consent' lawsuit brings to attention potential copyright issues related to the data used to train these models. There are also further unsettled copyright and intellectual property ownership questions regarding content generated by these models, e.g., new radiology images generated by DALL-E 2 in response to user's text prompts. Who owns the copyright to AI-generated content? Who should be held liable for any harm or loss it might cause? These issues become more complex when AI-generated content is based on copyrighted materials. Interestingly, Microsoft introduced a new section on AI services to its overall Services agreement effective September 30, 2023, in which it expanded the definition of "Your Content" to include "content that is generated by your use of our AI services".

Even when organizations can overcome these hurdles, one major challenge remains: focus and prioritization. In many boardrooms, executives are debating overwhelming lists of potential generative AI investments, only to deem them incomplete or outdated given the dizzying pace of innovation. These protracted debates are a waste of precious organizational energy—and time.

Setting the bar too high is setting up for failure. It's easy to get caught up, betting big on what seems like the greatest opportunity in the moment. But 12 months later, leaders often find themselves frustrated that they haven't seen results or feeling as if they've made a misplaced bet. Momentum and investments slow, further hindering progress.

Leading companies are forming a more pragmatic strategy that considers current capabilities, regulations, and barriers to adoption. Their CEOs and CFOs work together to enforce four guiding principles:

1. Pilot low-risk applications with a narrow focus first. Tomorrow's leaders are making no-regret moves to deliver savings and productivity enhancements in short order—at a time when they need it most. Gaining experience with currently available technology, they are testing and learning their way to minimum viable products in low-risk, repeatable use cases. These quick wins are typically in areas where they already have the right data, can create tight guardrails, and see a strong potential return on investment. Some, like call center and chatbot support, can improve the patient experience. However, given the current challenges around regulation and compliance, the most successful early initiatives are likely to be internally focused, such as billing or scheduling. Most importantly, executives prioritize initiatives by potential savings, value, and cost.
2. Decide to buy, partner, or build. CEOs will need to think about how to invest in different use cases based on availability of third-party technology and importance of the initiative
3. Funnel cost savings and experience into bigger bets. As the technology matures and the value becomes clear, companies that generate savings, accumulate experience, and build organizational buy-in today will be best positioned for the next wave of more sophisticated, transformative use cases. These include higher-risk clinical activities with a greater need for accuracy due to ethical and regulatory considerations, such as clinical decision support, as well as administrative activities that require third-party integration, such as prior authorization.
4. Remember generative AI isn't a strategy unto itself. To build a true competitive advantage, top CEOs and CFOs are selective and discerning, ensuring that every generative AI initiative reinforces and enables their overarching goals.

As with other emerging and rapidly developing technologies, the corresponding governing laws and regulations often lag and need some time to catch up. Some generative AI issues related to trust, safety, reliability, privacy, copyrights, and ownership are not yet fully settled (no definitive answers or solutions at the time of writing), but this does not mean they are unsurmountable. They will gradually get addressed over time as the technology evolves and matures and the laws, policies and regulatory frameworks surrounding its use start taking shape. Generative AI will play an increasingly important role in medicine and healthcare as it further evolves and gets better tailored to the unique settings and requirements of the medical domain. The coming years will see the introduction of new models specifically and comprehensively trained using corpora of quality evidence-based medical texts that sufficiently cover various clinical areas of specialism. These models will be of great help to healthcare professionals and their patients in the not-very-distant future. Rather than AI replacing humans (clinicians), we see it as "clinicians using AI" replacing "clinicians who do not use AI" in the following years

Chapter 9

Maintaining Human Touch in AI-driven Healthcare

Lessons from The Matrix

As we stand on the precipice of a new era in medicine, the rapid integration of Artificial Intelligence (AI) into healthcare has ushered in transformative changes. These changes promise improved diagnoses, streamlined processes, and personalized treatments. However, with this digital metamorphosis, there looms a significant challenge: ensuring that the heart and soul of medicine - the human touch - is not eclipsed by algorithms and codes. This chapter delves into the importance of preserving the irreplaceable human element in the ever-evolving landscape of AI-driven healthcare. We'll explore strategies to intertwine technology and human touch harmoniously, ensuring that patients receive not just effective but also compassionate care in the age of AI

"The Matrix" is a science fiction film that presents a future in which humanity is unknowingly trapped in a simulated reality, created by intelligent machines to distract humans while their bodies are used as an energy source. The protagonist, Neo, is initially a regular software engineer who feels there is something off about the world. He is drawn into a rebellion against the machines after learning the truth from Morpheus, a leader of the human resistance.

Throughout the film, Neo grapples with the nature of reality and his role in the fight against the AI that controls the Matrix. The film explores themes of human autonomy versus control by artificial intelligence, the nature of reality and illusion, and the struggle to reclaim genuine human experience from a manufactured, AI-driven world.

In the context of the chapter on "Maintaining Human Touch in AI-driven Healthcare," "The Matrix" serves as a metaphorical backdrop. It underscores the importance of preserving human elements - empathy, intuition, and ethical judgment - in the face of rapidly advancing AI technologies in healthcare. The film's narrative about humans striving to break free from the dominion of AI parallels concerns in modern healthcare about ensuring that AI aids, rather than replaces, the human touch in patient care. The movie's message about balancing technological advancement with the essence of human experience provides valuable insights for integrating AI into healthcare while maintaining a focus on patient-centered, empathetic care.

Balancing Efficiency with Empathy

The surge of Artificial Intelligence (AI) in medicine is revolutionizing patient care, from predictive algorithms and robotic surgeries to personalized treatment plans based on genomic data. These advancements promise a future where diseases might be diagnosed even before symptoms manifest, where treatments are tailored to the individual, and where medical errors are dramatically reduced. However, as we embrace these technological wonders, there emerges a pressing concern: How do we balance the unparalleled efficiency offered by AI with the deeply human quality of empathy that sits at the heart of healthcare?

Efficiency in medicine is not just about speed but accuracy. AI has demonstrated its prowess in both. For instance, machine learning algorithms can sift through medical images, identifying abnormalities often faster and, in some cases, more accurately than human counterparts. They can analyze vast datasets, drawing connections and patterns that might be inscrutable to the human eye. This means quicker diagnoses, more precise treatments, and, ultimately, better patient outcomes.

However, the essence of healthcare extends beyond diagnoses and treatments. It's about understanding a patient's fears, hopes, and concerns. It's about the reassuring touch of a nurse, the comforting words of a doctor, and the patience of a therapist. These are the intangibles that AI, at least in its current form, cannot replicate. Empathy, the ability to understand and share the feelings of another, remains a uniquely human trait. It's this empathy that often aids the healing process, providing patients with the psychological and emotional support they need.

So, how do we ensure that the integration of AI in medicine doesn't erode this bedrock of empathetic care?

Firstly, the role of AI should be seen as complementary to human medical practitioners, not a replacement. Doctors equipped with AI tools can potentially spend less time on manual, repetitive tasks, allowing them more quality time with patients. Instead of feeling rushed through appointments due to overwhelming caseloads, practitioners can utilize these moments to connect with patients, understand their concerns, and offer comfort.

Secondly, training programs for medical professionals should emphasize the irreplaceable value of human empathy. As AI takes on more diagnostic and analytical roles, the medical curriculum should pivot, focusing more on interpersonal skills, psychology, and patient communication. This will ensure that the next generation of healthcare providers retains the human touch, even in an AI-dominated landscape.

Lastly, AI developers should be encouraged to design systems with human-AI collaboration in mind. These systems should prioritize user-friendly interfaces, clear communication, and seamless integration into the patient-care process, ensuring that technology augments, rather than interrupts, the human connection.

The intersection of technology and humanity is no stranger to the cinematic world, and few films tackle it with as much depth and nuance as "The Matrix." At its core, the film challenges viewers to consider the consequences of surrendering our humanity to machines, a theme that resonates deeply with the current integration of AI in medicine.

AI's adoption in medicine brings with it efficiency and precision reminiscent of the intricate coding and systematic control found within the Matrix. Just as the simulated world offers a flawlessly efficient version of reality, AI promises a healthcare system with reduced errors, rapid diagnoses, and tailor-made treatments. Yet, the Matrix, for all its perfection, is void of genuine human experiences, emotions, and connections, mirroring concerns in today's medical landscape: the potential loss of empathy in the face of mechanized care.

Neo's journey from a passive recipient of the Matrix's constructed reality to an awakened challenger of the system symbolizes the necessary balance healthcare must strike. As Neo realizes the value of genuine human experience over the Matrix's sterile efficiency, so must healthcare professionals recognize the irreplaceable role of empathy, even in a technologically advanced setting. Just as the rebels in the film strive to reclaim their humanity from the machines, doctors, nurses, and therapists must ensure that the warmth of human touch isn't overshadowed by the cold precision of algorithms.

Moreover, Agent Smith's desire for control and efficiency, devoid of human imperfections, serves as a cautionary tale for medicine. While AI can streamline processes and reduce errors, a system entirely driven by efficiency, like Smith's vision, could strip away the compassion and understanding that lie at the heart of patient care. In the world of healthcare, every patient is an individual, not just a number in a system, much like each human outside the Matrix has a unique identity and value.

The rise of AI in medicine offers a tantalizing glimpse into a future of enhanced efficiency and precision. Yet, as we hurtle towards this future, we must carry with us the age-old values of empathy, compassion, and human connection. By consciously striving to balance efficiency with empathy, we can ensure that the healthcare of tomorrow is not just technologically advanced, but also deeply human. Weaving the lessons from "The Matrix" into the discourse on AI in medicine, it becomes evident that while technological advancement is inevitable and beneficial, it must be approached with caution. As Morpheus says, "It's the question that drives us." In medicine's case, the question is how to integrate AI without losing the essence of human connection. The answer lies in a conscious effort to balance efficiency with empathy, ensuring that as we step into the future, we carry with us the best of our humanity.

The Importance of Human Intuition and Expertise

In the modern era of healthcare, Artificial Intelligence (AI) stands as one of the most transformative forces. Its promises are many: early and precise diagnosis, tailored treatments, streamlined administrative tasks, and even the prediction of patient trajectories. Yet, for all its computational prowess, the human element of intuition and expertise remains paramount. As we incorporate AI into the healthcare landscape, it's crucial to recognize and uphold the unique value that human intuition and expertise bring to patient care.

Human intuition, honed over years of practice, education, and real-world experience, offers nuances that AI, in its current form, cannot entirely grasp. For example, while an AI algorithm might identify patterns in a patient's data suggesting a particular diagnosis, a seasoned doctor might sense, from a combination of verbal cues, body language, and subtle symptom presentations, that something else is at play. This intuitive leap, often built on years of clinical encounters, can lead to critical insights that might not yet be encoded into datasets and algorithms.

Furthermore, medical expertise extends beyond mere pattern recognition. It involves a deep understanding of the human body, disease processes, and the intricate balance of treatments, often acquired through extensive education, training, and patient interactions. A clinician's expertise encompasses not just knowledge but also the wisdom to apply this knowledge judiciously, factoring in the complexities of each patient's unique situation.

Moreover, the therapeutic relationship between a patient and their healthcare provider is built on trust. While AI can provide data, it cannot comfort a distressed patient, offer hope in the face of a challenging diagnosis, or understand the profound emotional and psychological dimensions of illness. Human expertise is not just about medical knowledge but also the ability to communicate, empathize, and build relationships.

It's also worth noting that AI, for all its advancements, is only as good as the data it's trained on. If there are biases in the data, AI can perpetuate and even amplify these biases, leading to skewed outcomes. Human expertise can act as a safeguard, identifying and correcting these biases, ensuring that care remains equitable and patient-centric.

However, this isn't to downplay AI's role in the future of medicine. Instead, it's a call for collaboration. The ideal healthcare landscape is one where AI assists and augments human intuition and expertise, not one where it seeks to replace it. By leveraging the strengths of both AI and human clinicians, we can move towards a healthcare system that is not only efficient and precise but also deeply compassionate and patient-focused.

The cinematic universe of "The Matrix" presents a world where artificial intelligence has not only matched but surpassed human capabilities, resulting in a simulated reality that keeps humanity dormant. This gripping narrative provides a thought-provoking backdrop against which we can explore the role of human intuition and expertise in the age of AI, especially in medicine.

At the heart of "The Matrix" lies a key conflict: the raw, computational efficiency of machines versus the deeply human qualities of intuition, emotion, and resilience. Neo, the film's protagonist, embodies this tension. Though the Matrix offers a flawless and controlled reality, it's Neo's inherent human intuition and the guidance of mentors like Morpheus that allow him to see beyond the simulation, question its veracity, and ultimately rebel against it.

Much like Neo's journey, AI in medicine can provide a structured, data-driven landscape. It can predict, analyze, and recommend with unparalleled speed. However, just as Neo relies on his instinct to navigate and challenge the Matrix, clinicians too rely on their intuition to interpret AI's recommendations, discerning when to follow them and when to lean on their expertise and judgment.

The Matrix, in its relentless quest for control and perfection, misses out on the nuances and unpredictabilities that define human existence. Similarly, while AI in medicine can manage vast amounts of data, it might miss the subtleties that a seasoned doctor, with years of experience, can detect. These subtleties can come in the form of a patient's demeanor, an inconsistency in their story, or a gut feeling that suggests looking beyond the obvious.

Morpheus's belief in the prophecy and his trust in Neo, despite the odds, exemplifies the irreplaceable value of human expertise and belief. In the realm of medicine, the relationship between a doctor and a patient, built on trust and years of expertise, is akin to this. An AI might predict outcomes based on data, but it's the doctor who, through experience and understanding, provides the necessary context, guidance, and reassurance.

Furthermore, the rebellion against the Matrix underscores the importance of questioning and challenging established norms. In the medical field, while AI can provide valuable insights, human experts must be vigilant, challenging AI's recommendations when necessary, ensuring that they align with the best interests of the patient.

"The Matrix" offers a powerful tale for the role of human intuition and expertise in AI-driven domains. As we integrate AI into medicine, the film serves as a reminder of the unique and irreplaceable qualities that humans bring to the table. Like Neo navigating the complexities of the Matrix, healthcare professionals must harness the power of AI while leaning on their innate human attributes to ensure the best outcomes for their patients. Remember that the heartbeat of healthcare is its human element. While we harness the power of AI to enhance patient care, the irreplaceable value of human intuition and expertise must remain at the forefront, guiding and shaping the future of medicine.

Patient-Centered Care in an Automated World

The surge of Artificial Intelligence (AI) in medicine is rapidly transforming the healthcare landscape. From diagnostic algorithms to predictive analytics and treatment optimization, AI offers a wealth of possibilities for enhancing patient care. But with this wave of automation, there arises an essential question: How can we ensure that healthcare remains patient-centered in an increasingly automated world?

Patient-centered care revolves around viewing the patient holistically, understanding not just their medical needs, but also their values, preferences, and socio-cultural background. It is about building a partnership with the patient, ensuring that their voice and choices play a pivotal role in the care they receive. In this ethos, every patient is more than just a collection of symptoms or a dataset, but a unique individual with emotions, hopes, fears, and dreams.

The introduction of AI in this setting is a double-edged sword. On one side, AI can tremendously enhance patient care. Algorithms can help diagnose diseases earlier, predict potential complications, tailor treatments to an individual's genetic makeup, and even optimize administrative tasks to reduce wait times. This can lead to more effective treatments, better outcomes, and increased patient satisfaction.

However, on the other side, there's a risk. If not integrated thoughtfully, AI might reduce patient interactions to mere transactions. Patients might feel they are being treated by machines rather than humans, leading to a sense of detachment and alienation. A diagnosis given by an algorithm, no matter how accurate, lacks the compassion and understanding a human doctor can offer.

To ensure that the rise of AI does not overshadow the importance of patient-centered care, several steps can be undertaken:

> Human-AI Collaboration: AI should be viewed as a tool to augment, not replace, human expertise. By offloading repetitive and data-intensive tasks to AI, doctors can have more time for meaningful interactions with patients, delving deeper into their concerns and building stronger doctor-patient relationships.
> Ethical Guidelines: As AI systems are integrated into healthcare, it's imperative to develop ethical guidelines ensuring they are used in ways that prioritize patient well-being and autonomy. This includes transparency about how AI is used and ensuring that patients always have the option to consult a human medical professional.
> Feedback Mechanisms: Incorporating feedback mechanisms where patients can share their experiences and concerns regarding AI-driven care can ensure that the technology is being used in ways that enhance, rather than hinder, the patient experience.
> Education and Communication: Patients should be educated about the role and limitations of AI in their care. Clear communication can help set realistic expectations and build trust.
> Interdisciplinary Approach: Integrating insights from fields such as psychology, sociology, and anthropology can ensure that AI tools are designed with a deep understanding of human behavior, needs, and socio-cultural nuances.

In the iconic world of "The Matrix," humans are imprisoned within a simulated reality, devoid of authentic experiences and true human connection, controlled by machines that prioritize efficiency and control over individual human essence. This dystopian tale provides a stark metaphor when considering the trajectory of AI in medicine and the imperative to maintain patient-centered care.

Just as inhabitants of the Matrix live within a meticulously constructed reality designed to keep them placated and oblivious, there's a potential danger in over-relying on AI in healthcare. If unchecked, patients could become mere data points within an algorithm, their unique experiences and stories overshadowed by the 'efficiency' of automated care. The Matrix serves as a cautionary tale of what can happen when individuality is lost in the face of automation.

Neo, the protagonist, seeks truth and authenticity in a world dominated by artificial constructs. Similarly, in an AI-driven healthcare environment, the onus is on medical professionals to ensure that care remains genuine and rooted in the realities and nuances of each patient's life. Just as Neo breaks free from the confines of the simulated reality to experience genuine human connections, medical care must transcend the binary codes of algorithms to truly connect with and understand patients.

The rebels in "The Matrix," led by Morpheus, fight to reclaim their humanity from the machines. This struggle can be likened to the challenge faced by healthcare providers: balancing the undeniable benefits of AI with the imperative to maintain a human touch in patient care. Morpheus's unwavering belief in the human spirit and its potential is a reminder of the innate human qualities - intuition, empathy, understanding - that machines cannot replicate. In medicine, these qualities form the bedrock of patient-centered care.

Agent Smith, with his vision of a 'perfect' world devoid of human unpredictability, is emblematic of a healthcare system that might prioritize efficiency at the cost of individual patient needs and emotions. While AI can streamline processes, a purely data-driven approach, much like Smith's vision for the Matrix, can strip away the very essence of patient-centered care.

Drawing inspiration from "The Matrix," the integration of AI in medicine should be approached with mindfulness. Just as the rebels seek a balance between the real and simulated worlds, healthcare must find its equilibrium, leveraging AI's capabilities without losing the patient's heart and soul in the process.

In conclusion, "The Matrix" offers profound insights into the challenges and responsibilities of introducing AI into sectors deeply rooted in human experience. In the quest for advanced and efficient healthcare, it serves as a poignant reminder of the irreplaceable value of genuine human connection and the importance of patient-centered care in an increasingly automated world. The challenge of integrating AI into medicine is not just a technical one but also a deeply human one. It's about harnessing the power of technology while ensuring that the core tenets of patient-centered care remain sacrosanct. With thoughtful implementation, it is entirely possible to create an automated world where healthcare is not just efficient but also deeply empathetic and patient-focused.

Chapter 10

Human -AI Collaboration

Lessons from the airline industry

On a cold January day in 2009, US Airways Flight 1549, piloted by Captain Chesley "Sully" Sullenberger and First Officer Jeffrey Skiles, faced an unprecedented crisis. Shortly after takeoff from New York's LaGuardia Airport, a flock of geese struck the aircraft, disabling both engines. In this critical moment, a blend of human expertise and advanced aviation technology culminated in what would be known as the "Miracle on the Hudson."

The Crisis Unfolds

As the engines failed, the Airbus A320 lost thrust, leaving the aircraft gliding over one of the world's busiest cities. The situation demanded an immediate response. While Captain Sully and First Officer Skiles assessed the scenario, the aircraft's advanced avionics, a product of sophisticated AI and automation technologies, provided crucial data on altitude, glide range, and potential landing sites.

Human Judgment and AI Assistance

Faced with limited options, the pilots considered returning to LaGuardia or diverting to Teterboro Airport. However, AI-assisted calculations and simulations indicated that reaching an airport was unlikely. At this juncture, the human decision-making process took center stage. Captain Sully, leveraging his extensive flying experience, made the critical call to ditch the plane in the Hudson River – a decision that AI alone couldn't have contextualized or executed.

The Role of AI in Crisis Management

The aircraft's AI systems played a pivotal role in assisting the crew during this emergency. Automated systems provided real-time data and calculations, which were essential for the pilots to understand their rapidly evolving situation. The AI also managed less critical flight tasks, allowing the pilots to focus exclusively on the emergency at hand.

The Ditching and Rescue

Executing a water landing with no engine power, Captain Sully relied on his flying skills and the aircraft's design to glide onto the river. The AI systems ensured that all on-board mechanisms functioned to minimize impact, while the structural integrity of the aircraft, enhanced by design innovations driven by AI and simulation data, played a crucial role in keeping the fuselage intact upon water impact.

All 155 passengers and crew members were safely evacuated onto the wings and rescued by nearby boats, marking a historic moment in aviation history.

Lessons in Human-AI Collaboration

The incident of Flight 1549 serves as a profound lesson in the power of human-AI collaboration. While AI provided critical data and managed complex calculations, it was Captain Sully's experience and decision-making *under pressure that led to the successful outcome. The event underscores the importance of human expertise in interpreting and acting upon AI-provided information, especially in unpredictable, high-stakes situations.*

Conclusion

The "Miracle on the Hudson" stands as a testament to the potential of human-AI collaboration in aviation. It highlights the indispensable value of human judgment and experience, complemented by the precision and efficiency of AI. This synergy between human and machine paves the way for a future in which AI enhances human capabilities, particularly in scenarios where every second counts.

In the dynamic world of aviation, ensuring safety is paramount. The evolution and adoption of Crew Resource Management (CRM) have played a crucial role in enhancing airline safety, marked by a profound shift in how crew members interact and make decisions during flights. This approach, focusing on human factors and effective teamwork, has been instrumental in reducing errors and managing emergency situations, such as the renowned "Miracle on the Hudson."

CRM emerged from an increasing awareness that human error, rather than technical failures, was often the root cause of aviation accidents. In the past, the hierarchical structure in cockpits and rigid communication protocols sometimes led to critical information being overlooked. CRM was developed to address these human factors by fostering a culture of open communication, teamwork, and decision-making based on collective input rather than rank.

Core Principles of CRM

The success of CRM lies in its core principles:

> ➢ Communication: Encouraging open and clear dialogue among crew members, regardless of rank, to ensure that vital information is shared and understood.

- Teamwork: Promoting collaboration and support among all crew members, recognizing that each has a vital role to play in ensuring the flight's safety.
- Decision-Making: Facilitating a more democratic process where decisions are made collectively, considering diverse perspectives and expertise.
- Situational Awareness: Maintaining a comprehensive understanding of the aircraft's environment, systems, and the potential impact of actions.
- Problem-Solving: Encouraging creative and effective solutions to unexpected situations, leveraging the collective skills of the crew.

The successful ditching of US Airways Flight 1549 in the Hudson River serves as a testament to the effectiveness of CRM. Captain Sully Sullenberger and First Officer Jeffrey Skiles worked in unison, maintaining open lines of communication, sharing vital information, and making joint decisions. This collaborative approach was crucial in assessing their situation, considering options, and choosing the best course of action under immense pressure. Here's how CRM principles were exemplified:

- Effective Communication: Immediately after the bird strike, there was clear and concise communication between Captain Sullenberger, First Officer Skiles, and air traffic control. This efficient exchange of information was crucial for quick decision-making.
- Teamwork and Leadership: Captain Sullenberger, as the pilot-in-command, took control of the aircraft while First Officer Skiles worked on the engine restart checklist. This division of duties under high-pressure circumstances reflected excellent teamwork and leadership, key tenets of CRM.
- Decision-Making Under Pressure: Captain Sullenberger made the critical decision to land on the Hudson River, considering the aircraft's altitude, the lack of nearby airports for a safe landing, and the densely populated areas of New York City. This

decision-making process, under extreme pressure, is a hallmark of CRM training.
- ➤ Resource Utilization: The crew utilized all available resources, including each other's expertise, the aircraft's remaining glide capabilities, and even input from air traffic control, to manage the crisis.
- ➤ Situational Awareness: Maintaining situational awareness was crucial. The crew was constantly aware of the aircraft's altitude, speed, and potential landing sites, which guided their decision to ditch in the river.

Over the years, CRM has evolved to include all aspects of flight operations, extending beyond the cockpit to include cabin crews, maintenance personnel, and ground staff. This comprehensive approach ensures that safety is a collective responsibility, shared by all who contribute to the operation of a flight.

Key to the success of CRM is ongoing training and real-world application. Simulation-based training, workshops, and continuous learning opportunities are integral, helping crew members develop and refine their CRM skills. Airlines around the world now incorporate CRM principles into their standard training programs, recognizing their critical role in maintaining safety.

CRM has revolutionized the aviation industry, significantly reducing accidents and incidents attributed to human error. It has fostered a culture where safety is paramount, and effective teamwork is the norm. The principles of CRM, highlighted in incidents like the "Miracle on the Hudson," continue to be a guiding force in aviation, ensuring that safety remains at the forefront of every flight operation.

As the healthcare industry navigates the uncharted territories of Artificial Intelligence, drawing parallels with the aviation industry's approach to safety and coordination is not only insightful but also increasingly necessary. The aviation industry's Crew Resource Management (CRM) has been a cornerstone of its safety culture. CRM in aviation focuses on effective teamwork, communication, and decision-making to ensure safety. Translating this to healthcare, especially in the context of AI, means fostering an environment where technology complements human expertise, enhancing patient care and clinical outcomes.

Clinical Team Coordination (CTC)©

Hospital XYZ, a pioneer in adopting AI for patient diagnostics, encountered challenges that highlighted the need for a CRM approach. Their AI system, designed to assist in diagnosing complex diseases, was initially met with enthusiasm. However, it soon became apparent that reliance on AI without proper team coordination and understanding could lead to errors. A significant incident occurred when an AI-recommended treatment for a rare condition was questioned by a junior doctor but ultimately not reviewed by senior staff, leading to a misdiagnosis. This incident underscored the potential dangers of uncoordinated AI integration in healthcare settings.

The integration of AI in healthcare, much like the introduction of advanced avionics in aviation, requires a well-thought-out strategy to ensure safety. The interaction between humans and AI systems in dynamic and high-stakes environments like healthcare is complex and can lead to new types of errors. The author's Clinical Team Coordination (CTC)© approach, akin to aviation's CRM, provides a structured way to manage the complexities of AI in a clinical environment. It emphasizes the critical balance between human expertise and technological advancement. As we embrace the AI era in healthcare, the CTC model stands as a beacon, guiding us towards a future where patient safety remains paramount, and AI serves as a tool for enhancement, not a replacement for human judgment.

Drawing from the aviation industry's CRM, the author introduced CTC© with the following components:

> ➢ Improved Communication: Like CRM's emphasis on clear, assertive communication in the cockpit, CTC promoted open

dialogue among healthcare teams regarding AI decisions. This ensured that AI recommendations were scrutinized and validated, enhancing decision-making processes.
- ➤ Defined Roles and Decision Hierarchies: Clear role definitions were established, underscoring that AI tools were supports, not replacements, for clinical judgment. This helped maintain the delicate balance between human expertise and AI assistance.
- ➤ Training for Effective Human-AI Interaction: Similar to pilot training on automated systems, healthcare staff received training on effectively interpreting and using AI tools, fostering a deeper understanding and better management of AI in clinical settings.
- ➤ Non-punitive Error Reporting: Inspired by aviation's safety reporting systems, a similar mechanism was implemented for AI-related errors. This fostered a culture of continuous learning and improvement, crucial for evolving AI systems.

A compelling example of the application of CTC principles is the story of XYZ Hospital's Emergency Department and their handling of a complex medical emergency using AI, guided by the principles of CTC. XYZ Hospital faced a critical situation when a patient, Mr. Thompson, arrived experiencing severe chest pain and signs of a stroke. The situation was complex, as the symptoms pointed to multiple potential diagnoses. The medical team decided to utilize their AI diagnostic tool for a more accurate assessment.

The way the medical team at XYZ Hospital managed this crisis with the help of AI, while adhering to CTC principles, is instructive:

1. Effective Communication: The team maintained open communication lines, with each member providing insights based on their expertise. This collaborative approach was crucial in interpreting the AI tool's findings.
2. Defined Roles and Collaborative Decision-Making: The AI system suggested a rare combination of ailments, which the team initially found surprising. However, Dr. Lee, the leading physician, encouraged the team to discuss the AI's findings critically,

combining their medical knowledge with the AI's data-driven insights.
3. Training and Familiarity with AI Tools: The medical staff's training in using the AI system efficiently allowed them to understand and trust its recommendations, while also knowing its limitations.
4. Error Reporting and Feedback Mechanism: The hospital had a system for reporting discrepancies in AI recommendations. This non-punitive approach encouraged team members to voice concerns and learn from each interaction with the AI system.
5. Situational Awareness and Human Oversight: The team was aware that AI tools are aids, not decision-makers. Dr. Lee, understanding the gravity of the situation, used the AI's analysis as one component of a broader diagnostic strategy.

The AI's recommendation, combined with the team's expertise, led to the identification of a rare co-occurrence of conditions that required immediate and specific intervention. Mr. Thompson's life was saved due to the timely and accurate diagnosis. This case demonstrates the transformative impact of Clinical Team Coordination in healthcare, especially in scenarios where AI plays a crucial role. It highlights how effective communication, collaborative decision-making, continuous learning, and maintaining human oversight can ensure that AI in medicine serves as a powerful tool for enhancing patient care, much like how CRM revolutionized safety in aviation. The CTC model is more than a guideline; it's a beacon for navigating the intricate interplay of AI in the complex and high-stakes field of medicine.

The objectives of CTC training prior to implementing AI in Healthcare, include:

➢ Enhance understanding of human-technology collaboration principles and their importance in optimizing healthcare delivery.
➢ Develop skills for effective teamwork with AI and other technologies in clinical settings.
➢ Improve communication and coordination between team members and technology systems.

➤ Foster a culture of trust and acceptance of technology as a valuable partner in healthcare.
➤ Reduce errors and improve patient outcomes through effective human-technology interaction.

The components of the program include:

Introduction to Human-Technology Collaboration in Healthcare:

- Demystifying AI and other healthcare technologies and their roles in clinical workflows.
- Exploring the potential benefits and challenges of human-technology collaboration.
- Understanding the importance of clear roles and responsibilities for both humans and technology.

Communication for Effective Collaboration:

- Active listening and assertive communication with technology systems.
- Providing clear instructions and feedback to AI algorithms.
- Interpreting and questioning technology outputs critically.
- Effective communication within the clinical team regarding technology-based decisions.

Teamwork and Coordination Strategies:

- Defining roles and responsibilities for team members and technology in different clinical scenarios.
- Developing standard operating procedures for integrating technology into workflows.
- Leading and fostering open communication and collaboration within the team.
- Addressing conflicts and managing resistance to change related to technology implementation.

Situational Awareness and Decision-Making:

- Maintaining awareness of technology capabilities and limitations during decision-making.
- Recognizing and mitigating potential biases and errors in technology outputs.
- Balancing reliance on technology with independent clinical judgment and expertise.
- Escalating critical situations and effectively requesting human intervention when needed.

Building Trust and Acceptance of Technology:

- Addressing concerns and anxieties about AI and other technologies within the team.
- Highlighting positive examples of successful human-technology collaboration in healthcare.
- Promoting ongoing learning and upskilling to adapt to evolving technology landscape.
- Engaging team members in the selection and evaluation of healthcare technologies.

Scenario-Based Learning and Simulation:

- Role-playing exercises and simulations to apply CTC principles in realistic clinical scenarios.
- Practicing communication and collaboration with simulated AI systems.
- Debriefing and feedback for individual and team learning and improvement.

Next Steps and Continuous Improvement:

- Developing an action plan for implementing CTC best practices in your workplace.

- Identifying opportunities for ongoing training and support for human-technology collaboration.
- Establishing feedback mechanisms and channels for continuous improvement of CTC practices.

CTC training fosters the missing link between the immense potential of AI and its successful integration into real-world medical practice. Here's why:

- Optimizes teamwork and communication: CTC equips healthcare teams to seamlessly interact with AI systems, providing clear instructions, interpreting outputs critically, and navigating challenges of joint decision-making. This seamless interaction prevents friction and maximizes the combined strengths of humans and AI.
- Minimizes risk and error: With proper understanding of AI capabilities and limitations, CTC empowers healthcare professionals to identify and mitigate potential biases, errors, and misinterpretations in AI outputs. This safeguards patient outcomes and builds trust in the technology.
- Builds trust and acceptance: Open communication and collaboration fostered by CTC training address anxieties and concerns surrounding AI. By showcasing successful integrations and promoting ongoing learning, CTC paves the way for acceptance and active participation in the AI revolution.
- Boosts efficiency and accuracy: Through CTC, teams learn to efficiently leverage AI's strengths in data analysis, pattern recognition, and automation. This streamlines workflows, reduces tedious tasks, and potentially allows for more accurate diagnoses and personalized treatment plans.
- Empowers clinicians and promotes ownership: CTC training doesn't simply replace humans with machines; it empowers clinicians to become effective collaborators with AI. This shared ownership fosters a sense of agency and encourages active participation in shaping the future of healthcare.

CTC training is not just a nice-to-have, it's a critical cornerstone for the successful implementation of AI in medicine. By bridging the gap between humans and technology, CTC ensures safe, effective, and ultimately transformative healthcare for all. Investing in CTC training is an investment in the future, paving the way for a collaborative, AI-powered healthcare ecosystem that prioritizes both efficiency and human connection.

Remember, AI may hold the key to unlocking remarkable improvements in healthcare, but only when paired with the human skill, judgment, and empathy cultivated through programs like CTC. Only then can we truly unlock the transformative potential of AI in medicine.

Chapter 11

Ambient Intelligence in Healthcare

Sarah, 78, lives alone in her independent living apartment, managing her early-stage Alzheimer's with medication and regular check-ins from her daughter, Emily. One night, Sarah takes a tumble in her kitchen, hitting her head and disorienting herself. Fear and confusion cloud her memory, preventing her from calling for help.

Sensors embedded in Sarah's floor register the sudden fall, triggering an alert on Emily's smartphone. The smart lights in Sarah's kitchen automatically switch on, bathing the room in a soft glow to calm her agitation. A familiar voice from the smart speaker reassures Sarah, gently prompting her to sit down and activate her emergency bracelet.

Meanwhile, in the background, the ambient intelligence (AmI) network hums:

- *Sarah's wearable health tracker detects an elevated heart rate and transmits the data to her doctor, who is alerted on their device.*
- *Smart cameras in the hallway capture footage of Sarah's fall, which is analyzed by an AI algorithm to assess the severity of the injury.*
- *The AI system coordinates a response, contacting emergency services and sending Emily directions to her mother's apartment.*

By the time Emily arrives, paramedics are already on the scene. Sarah, though shaken, is unharmed thanks to the swift intervention of the AmI network. The doctor, armed with data from Sarah's fall and real-time health readings, can make informed decisions about her treatment.

The impact of AmI goes beyond the immediate crisis:

- *Sarah regains confidence and independence, knowing her AmI guardian is always watching over her.*
- *Emily finds peace of mind, knowing her mother is safe and receiving immediate care in case of emergencies.*
- *Sarah's doctor can monitor her condition more effectively, adjusting medication and care plans based on real-time data.*

As illustrated in the preceding case of Sarah, Ambient Intelligence (AmI) refers to electronic environments that are sensitive and responsive to the presence of people. In the context of healthcare, it involves the use of embedded and interconnected devices and systems to collect, analyze, and interpret data to provide personalized and adaptive healthcare services. This chapter delves into the concept of Ambient Intelligence in healthcare, exploring its potential benefits, applications, and challenges. We will examine how Ambient Intelligence can enhance patient care, improve health outcomes, and transform healthcare delivery, across healthcare and in home-based care settings. As leaders at the forefront of responsible AI in healthcare, we must understand AmI's potential, navigate its ethical complexities, and harness its power to create a future where technology cares, not just cures. In hospital spaces, early applications could soon enable more efficient clinical workflows and improved patient safety in intensive care units and operating rooms. In daily living spaces, ambient intelligence could prolong the independence of older individuals and improve the management of individuals with a chronic disease by understanding everyday behavior.

Take, for instance, the recent announcement by the US National Highway Traffic Safety Administration (NHTSA) exploring AmI's potential in combating drunk driving. Imagine cars equipped with sensors that detect signs of intoxication through speech analysis, breath tests, or even eye-tracking. Such systems could not only prevent a driver from taking the wheel under the influence but also trigger alerts to notify authorities or loved ones. While ethical concerns around data privacy and false positives remain, the potential to save lives through this proactive approach is undeniable.

Across the Atlantic, in the UK, the National Health Service (NHS) is piloting a program that utilizes AmI in an unexpected way: monitoring energy usage in people's homes. Smart meters and connected appliances track kettle and fridge usage, identifying patterns that might indicate health risks like dehydration or medication non-adherence. This initiative aims to reduce avoidable hospital admissions by providing timely interventions like food deliveries or cleaning services. While some raise concerns about intrusive surveillance, the project's goal is to provide early intervention for vulnerable individuals, potentially preventing hospital admissions and fostering healthy living habits.

This chapter explores how ambient, contactless sensors, in addition to contact-based wearable devices, can illuminate two health-critical environments: hospitals and daily living spaces.

Hospital spaces

In 2018, approximately 7.4% of the US population required an overnight hospital stay. In the same year, 17 million admission episodes were reported by the National Health Service (NHS) in the UK. Yet, healthcare workers are often overworked, and hospitals understaffed and resource-limited. We discuss a number of hospital spaces in which ambient intelligence may have an important role in improving the quality of healthcare delivery, the productivity of clinicians, and business operations. These improvements could be of great assistance during healthcare crises, such as pandemics, during which time hospitals encounter a surge of patients20.

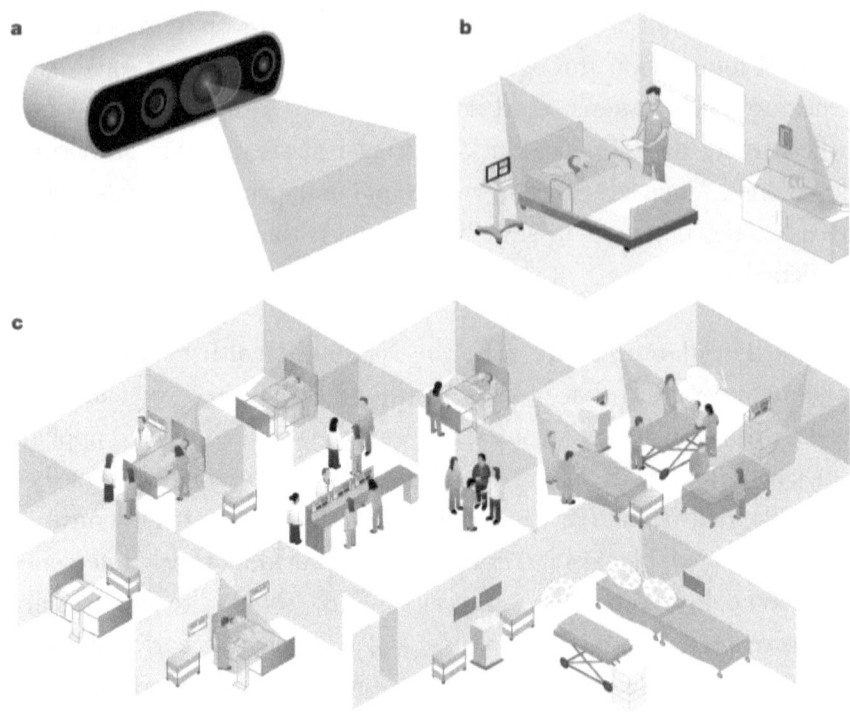

Ambient intelligence for hospitals: a, Commercial ambient sensor for which the coverage area is shown in green (that is, the field of view of visual sensors and range for acoustic and radio sensors). **b**, Sensors deployed inside a patient room can capture conversations and the physical motions of patients, clinicians and visitors. **c**, Sensors can be deployed throughout a hospital.

ICU's

One promising use case of ambient intelligence in ICUs is the computer-assisted monitoring of patient mobilization. ICU-acquired weaknesses are a common neuromuscular impairment in critically ill patients, potentially leading to a twofold increase in one-year mortality rate and 30% higher hospital costs. Early patient mobilization could reduce the relative incidence of ICU-acquired weaknesses by 40%. Currently, the standard mobility assessment is through direct, in-person observation, although its use is limited by cost impracticality, observer bias and human error. Proper measurement requires a nuanced understanding of patient movements. For example, localized wearable devices can detect pre-ambulation manoeuvres (for example, the transition from sitting to standing), but are unable to detect external assistance or interactions with the physical space (for example, sitting on chair versus bed). Contactless, ambient sensors could provide the continuous and nuanced understanding needed to accurately measure patient mobility in ICUs.

Operating Rooms

nother early application is the control of hospital infections. Worldwide, more than 100 million patients are affected by hospital-acquired (that is, nosocomial) infections each year, with up to 30% of patients in ICUs experiencing a nosocomial infection. Proper compliance with hand hygiene protocols is one of the most effective methods of reducing the frequency of nosocomial infections. However, measuring compliance remains challenging. In a pioneering study, researchers installed depth sensors above wall-mounted dispensers across an entire hospital unit. A deep-learning algorithm achieved an accuracy of 75% at measuring compliance for 351 handwashing events during one hour. During the same time period, an in-person observer was 63% accurate, while a proximity algorithm (for example, RFID) was only 18% accurate.

One study used cameras, microphones and accelerometers to monitor 22 patients in ICUs, with and without delirium, over 7 days. The study found significantly fewer head motions of patients who were delirious compared with patients who were not. Future studies could leverage this technology to detect delirium sooner and provide researchers with a deeper understanding of how patient mobilization affects mortality, length of stay and patient recovery.

Worldwide, more than 230 million surgical procedures are undertaken annually with up to 14% of patients experiencing an adverse event. This percentage could be reduced through quicker surgical feedback, such as more frequent coaching of technical skill, which could reduce the number of errors by 50%. Currently, the skills of a surgeon are assessed by peers and supervisors, despite being time-consuming, infrequent and subjective. Ambient cameras are an unobtrusive alternative. One study trained a convolutional neural network to track a needle driver in prostatectomy videos. Using peer-evaluation as the reference standard, the algorithm categorized 12 surgeons into high- and low-skill groups with an accuracy of 92%. A different study used videos from ten cholecystectomy procedures to reconstruct the trajectories of instruments during surgery and linked them to technical ratings by expert surgeons.

In the operating room, ambient intelligence is not limited to endoscopic videos. Another example is the surgical count—a process of counting used objects to prevent objects being accidentally retained inside the patient. Currently, dedicated staff time and effort are required to visually and verbally count these objects. Owing to attention deficit and insufficient team communication, it is possible for the human-adjudicated count to incorrectly label an object as returned when it is actually missing. Automated counting systems, in particular, could assist surgical teams

Other healthcare spaces

Clinicians spend up to 35% of their time on medical documentation tasks, taking valuable time away from patients. Currently, physicians perform documentation during or after each patient visit. Some providers use medical scribes to alleviate this burden, resulting in 0.17 more patients seen per hour and 0.21 more relative value units per patient (that is, insurer reimbursement). However, scribes are expensive to train and have high turnover. Ambient microphones could perform a similar task to that of medical scribes. Medical dictation software is an alternative, but is traditionally limited to the post-visit report. In one study, researchers trained a deep-learning model on 14,000h of outpatient audio from 90,000 conversations between patients and physicians. The model demonstrated a word-level transcription accuracy of 80%, suggesting it may be better than the 76% accuracy of medical scribes. In terms of clinical utility, one medical provider found that microphones attached to eyeglasses reduced time spent on documentation from 2 h to 15 min and doubled the time spent with patients.

Daily living spaces

Humans spend a considerable portion of time at home. Around the world, the population is ageing. Not only will this increase the amount of time spent at home, but it will also increase the importance of independent living, chronic disease management, physical rehabilitation and mental health of older individuals in daily living spaces.

Elderly living spaces and ageing

By 2050, the world's population aged 65 years or older will increase from 700 million to 1.5 billion. Activities of daily living (ADLs), such as bathing, dressing and eating, are critical to the well-being and independence of this population. Impairment of one's ability to perform ADLs is associated with a twofold increase in falling risk and up to a fivefold increase in one-year mortality rate. Earlier detection of impairments could provide an opportunity to provide timely clinical care11, potentially improving the ability to perform ADL by a factor of two74. Currently, ADLs are measured through self-reported questionnaires or manual grading by caregivers, despite the fact that these measurements are infrequent, biased and subjective. Alternatively, wearable devices (such as accelerometers or electrocardiogram sensors) can track not only ADLs, but also heart rate, glucose level and respiration rate. However, wearable devices are unable to discern whether a patient received ADL assistance—a key component of ADL evaluations. Contactless, ambient sensors could potentially identify these clinical nuances while detecting a greater range of activities. In one of the first studies of its kind, researchers installed a depth and thermal sensor inside the bedroom of an older individual and observed 1,690 activities during 1 month, including 231 instances of caregiver assistance. A convolutional neural network1 was 86% accurate at detecting assistance.

Another application for the independent living of older individuals is fall detection. Approximately 29% of community-dwelling adults fall at least once a year. Laying on the floor for more than one hour after a fall is correlated with a fivefold increase in 12-month mortality. Furthermore, the fear of falling—associated with depression and lower quality of life—can be reduced due to the perceived safety benefit of fall-detection systems. For decades, researchers developed fall-detection systems with wearable devices and contactless ambient sensors. A systematic review found that wearable devices detected falls with 96% accuracy while ambient sensors were 97% accurate.

Ambient AI at the point of care

Ambient AI promises a second coming for technology at the point of care enabling EHR systems to elegantly work for providers in the background, in natural workflows and "in conversation," versus requiring the provider and patients to step aside, waste time, and "feed the beasts" of legacy transactional systems. Ambient AI will prove as the key foundation to improving the patient experience, reducing provider burnout, improving documentation quality, while also helping to boost patient access and provider productivity.

Perhaps the hottest subsegment of ambient AI innovation is in the area of what people refer to as the "voice" space. Voice solutions have been widely adopted in healthcare for decades now. Most are familiar with the process: a physician sees a patient, steps aside (perhaps in the hallway), and then takes several precious minutes to verbatim speak out the notes (we call this typing with your tongue). This approach is a dictation workflow, and I certainly wouldn't consider it ambient. In the future, sensors placed throughout the care environment (or present with or on the provider) will process provider-patient conversations as they unfold in real-time, using speech recognition and natural language processing technology in the background to produce high-quality documentation. This approach places note data right where it belongs, without burdening the provider or interrupting the provider-patient connection. In fact, companies like Augmedix has such a solution in the market.

Ambient AI solutions will be merging into video calls with your provider teams, documenting, translating, and surfacing insights as needed. When you reach a call center to schedule your next appointment, voice markers of depression, anxiety, and other metadata will be collected to help determine next steps and manage your care and experience.

Chronic disease management

Gait analysis, vital for treating conditions like cerebral palsy and Parkinson's disease, is evolving from lab-based methods to wearable and contactless technologies. This shift allows for more frequent and accurate monitoring in natural settings. For example, studies using depth sensors for Parkinson's patients showed promising results in tracking knee movements. Additionally, combining different sensor modalities, like microphones and wearables, has shown improved gait detection accuracy. These advancements in ambient intelligence technologies are pivotal for healthcare leaders to consider, as they offer enhanced patient care through more precise and convenient monitoring methods.

Mental Health

In the context of mental health, ambient intelligence offers innovative approaches for diagnosing and treating conditions like depression, anxiety, and bipolar disorder. Traditional methods, such as self-reported questionnaires and clinical evaluations, often fall short due to infrequency and bias. Ambient sensors, however, promise continuous and cost-effective symptom screening. Studies using machine learning with audio, video, and movement data have shown high accuracy in detecting conditions like schizophrenia. In psychotherapy, ambient sensors could provide more efficient, higher-quality data for research, potentially leading to better treatment outcomes. This evolving field holds significant promise for improving mental health care, though further research is needed for broader application and validation.

Social and ethical considerations

Privacy

Trustworthiness of ambient intelligence systems is critical to achieve the potential of this technology. Ambient sensors, by design, continuously observe the environment and can uncover new information about how physical human behaviors influence the delivery of healthcare. For example, sensors can measure vital signs from a distance. While convenient, such knowledge could potentially be used to infer private medical conditions. As citizens worldwide are becoming more sensitive to mass data collection, there are growing concerns over confidentiality, sharing and retention of this information. It is therefore essential to co-develop this technology with privacy and security in mind, not only in terms of the technology itself but also in terms of a continuous involvement of all stakeholders during the development.

There are a number of existing and emerging privacy-preserving techniques. One method is to de-identify data by removing the identities of the individuals. Another method is data minimization, which minimizes data capture, transport and human bycatch. An ambient system could pause when a hospital room is unoccupied by a patient. However, even if data are de-identified, it may be possible to re-identify an individual. Super-resolution techniques can partially reverse the effects of face blurring and dimensionality reduction techniques, potentially enabling re-identification. This suggests that data should remain on-device to reduce the risk of unauthorized access and re-identification.

Legal and social complexities will inevitably arise. There are documented examples in which companies were required to provide data from ambient speakers and cameras to law enforcement. Although these devices were located inside potential crime scenes, this raises the question at what point incidental findings outside the crime scene, such as inadvertent confessions, should be disclosed. Related to data sharing, some healthcare organizations have shared patient information with third parties such as data brokers. To mitigate this, patients should proactively request healthcare providers to use privacy-preserving practices. Additionally, clinicians and technologists must collaborate with critical stakeholders (for example, patients, family or caregivers), legal experts and policymakers to develop governance frameworks for ambient systems.

Fairness

Ambient intelligence will interact with large patient populations, potentially several orders of magnitude larger than the reach of current clinicians. This compels us to scrutinize the fairness of ambient systems. Fairness is a complex and multi-faceted topic, discussed previously. Here, we two aspects of algorithmic fairness as examples: dataset bias and model performance.

Labelled datasets are the foundation of most machine-learning systems. However, medical datasets have been biased, even before deep learning. These biases can adversely affect clinical outcomes for certain populations. If an individual is missing specific attributes, whether owing to data-collection constraints or societal factors, algorithms could misinterpret their entire record, resulting in higher levels of predictive error. One method for identifying bias is to analyze model performance across different groups. In one study, error rates varied across ethnic groups when predicting 30-day psychiatric readmission rates. A more rigorous method could test for equal sensitivity and equal positive-predictive value. However, equal model performance may not produce equal clinical outcomes, as some populations may have inherent physiological differences.

Transparency

Ambient intelligence can uncover insights about how healthcare delivery is influenced by human behavior. These discoveries may surprise some researchers, in which case, clinicians and patients need to trust the findings before using them. Instead of opaque, black-box models, ambient intelligence systems should provide interpretable results that are predictive, descriptive and relevant. This can aid in the challenging task of acquiring stakeholder buy-in, as technical illiteracy and model opacity can stagnate efforts to use ambient intelligence in healthcare. Transparency is not limited to the algorithm. Dataset transparency—a detailed trace of how a dataset was designed, collected and annotated—would allow for specific precautions to be taken for future applications, such as training human annotators or revising the inclusion and exclusion criteria of a study. Formal guidelines on transparency, such as the Transparent Reporting of a multivariable prediction model for Individual Prognosis Or Diagnosis (TRIPOD)[14] statement, are actively being developed. Another tool is the use of model cards, which are short analyses that benchmark the algorithm across different populations and outline evaluation procedures.

Centuries of medical practice led to a knowledge explosion, fueling unprecedented advances in human health. Breakthroughs in artificial intelligence and low-cost, contactless sensors have given rise to an ambient intelligence that can potentially improve the physical execution of healthcare delivery. Preliminary results from hospitals and daily living spaces confirm the richness of information gained through ambient sensing. This extraordinary opportunity to illuminate the dark spaces of healthcare requires computer scientists, clinicians and medical researchers to work closely with experts from law, ethics and public policy to create trustworthy ambient intelligence systems for healthcare.

---

[14] https://www.acpjournals.org/doi/10.7326/m14-0697#:~:text=The%20TRIPOD%20Statement%20aims%20to,TRIPOD%20explanation%20and%20elaboration%20document.

Chapter 12

Green AI in Healthcare

The 'why' of Green AI in healthcare is straightforward - sustainability. The health care sector, in its pursuit of saving lives, has a considerable environmental footprint. In fact, it is estimated that the health care sector accounts for around 4 percent of global greenhouse gas emissions, and according to Health Care Without Harm, if the global health care sector were a country, it would be the fifth-largest greenhouse gas emitter on the planet. Healthcare stands at a crossroads. While AI promises revolutionary diagnoses, personalized treatments, and streamlined workflows, its growing shadow falls upon the environment. Energy-hungry algorithms, sprawling data centers, and mountains of electronic waste – the price of progress can be steep. This is where Green AI steps in, offering a symbiotic solution: enhancing care while minimizing environmental impact.

AI systems, particularly those based on deep learning, require substantial computational resources, leading to significant energy consumption and carbon emissions. According to one study by the University of Massachusetts, training AI models to do Natural Language Processing (NLP), can produce the carbon dioxide equivalent of 5X the lifetime emissions of the American car, or the equivalent of 300 round-trip flights between San Francisco and New York. This example of CO_2 emissions from AI is stunning and disturbing. It is a wake-up call for us all. As the use of AI in healthcare expands, so does its environmental footprint. Therefore, there is a pressing need to ensure that the benefits of AI do not come at the expense of our planet. Green AI is a necessity, not a luxury. Unmitigated, the carbon footprint of AI in healthcare could soar, negating the very progress it promises. Moreover, sustainability is not just about protecting the environment; it's about protecting vulnerable populations disproportionately affected by pollution and climate change. Green AI in healthcare, therefore, is not just an environmental imperative, but an ethical one.

As health care leaders executives, we need to ask for the information that is not being collected at this time by your AI teams. Without data about your AI carbon footprint, you may be creating a surprise reputational risk for the company once information about your carbon footprint becomes public. Without data about the potential environmental impact of your future AI projects, you cannot fully evaluate your investment in any project. Now more than ever, the impact of AI on CO_2 emissions needs to be a key element in your decision-making process.

Interestingly, Canada's Montreal Institute for Learning Algorithms has recently released a tool designed to estimate how much carbon is produced in training machine learning models. This particular tool is a small step in the right direction. At this moment, few other tools exist. It will be incumbent upon your AI teams to either use other tools or create their own to address the board's questions about environmental impact. As environmental sustainability becomes more important, we need a lot more information about the impact our company is having. We need to track and report on what is happening inside our company as it relates to environmental sustainability. Younger clinicians who are coming of age now and starting to work in health care are passionate about the climate crisis. They see it for what it is, which is an existential threat and the greatest public health threat we face on the planet. There's a very powerful argument that phasing out fossil fuels will also be good for people's health. So there's a very strong health-based reason to address the climate crisis.

Younger Americans—millennials and adults in Generation Z—stand out in a new Pew Research Center survey, particularly for their high levels of engagement with the issue of climate change. Compared with older adults, Gen Zers and millennials are talking more about the need for action on climate change. Among social media users, they are seeing more climate change content online, and they are doing more to get involved with the issue through activities such as volunteering and attending rallies and protests.

AI has the potential to produce significant and impactful carbon emissions. AI also has the potential to offset or reduce those carbon emissions. Healthcare organizations should consider allying themselves with any cloud provider that is committed to reducing their carbon footprint, thereby reducing their own. Instead of focusing on major internal projects to reduce environmental impact, it's possible to shift a company's AI training and processing to a data center cloud provider that can do that for you. For example:

- Google's DeepMind division has developed AI that teaches itself to minimize the use of energy to cool Google's data centers. As a result, Google reduced its data center energy requirements by 35%. Google's public cloud offering is called Google Cloud Platform.
- Microsoft has committed to be carbon negative by 2030. Microsoft also runs massive public data centers (cloud offerings) under the name Microsoft Azure.
- Amazon has a long-term goal of powering its global infrastructure using 100% renewable energy. This includes its cloud platform AWS.

AI can be a net positive contributor to environmental sustainability in many industries. Here are some examples:

In agriculture, AI can transform production by better monitoring and managing environmental conditions and crop yields. AI can help reduce both fertilizer and water, all while improving crop yields.

In energy, AI can use deep predictive capabilities and intelligent grid systems to manage the demand and supply of renewable energy. By more accurately predicting weather patterns, AI can optimize efficiency, cutting costs, and unnecessary carbon pollution generation.

In transportation, AI can help reduce traffic congestion, improve the transport of cargo (supply chain logistics), and enable more and more autonomous driving capability. AI will eventually help with the "last mile" delivery problem and reduce the need for delivery vehicles. AI can help businesses with demand forecasting, helping to reduce the amount of transport needed.

In water resource management, AI can help reduce or eliminate waste while lowering costs and lessening environmental impact. AI-driven localized weather forecasting will help reduce water usage.

In manufacturing, AI can help reduce waste and energy use in production facilities. Robotics can enable better precision. AI can design more efficient systems.

In facilities management, AI can help recycle heat within buildings and maximize the efficiency of heating and cooling. AI can help optimize energy use in buildings by tracking the number of people in a room or predicting the availability of renewable energy sources.

In materials science, AI can help researchers find new materials for solar panels, for turning heat back into useful electricity and to help find absorbent materials as components of CO_2 scrubbers (taking CO_2 out of the atmosphere.)

Artificial Intelligence (AI) can contribute to environmental sustainability in healthcare in several ways:

Three areas where AI is likely to have an impact on environmental sustainability:

1. Optimizing Resource Utilization:

Energy Efficiency: AI can analyze and optimize energy consumption in hospitals, predicting demand and adjusting operations accordingly. Think smart thermostats, AI-powered HVAC systems, and energy-efficient medical equipment.

Waste Reduction: AI can identify and streamline processes to minimize medical waste, optimize supply chains, and predict equipment maintenance needs, reducing both waste production and resource consumption.

Resource Management: AI can analyze patient data and medical history to personalize treatment plans, reducing unnecessary testing, medication overuse, and hospital stays.

2. Empowering Green Innovations:

Renewable Energy: AI can integrate renewable energy sources into healthcare infrastructure, predicting energy demand and managing microgrids to maximize reliance on sustainable energy.

Green Logistics: AI can optimize patient transportation, ambulance dispatch, and medical supply delivery, reducing transportation emissions and fuel consumption.

Telemedicine and Remote Care: AI-powered telemedicine platforms can reduce the need for physical travel, minimizing transportation emissions and the environmental impact of healthcare facilities.

3. Driving Sustainable Development:

Predictive Maintenance: AI can predict equipment failures and schedule preventive maintenance, extending the lifespan of medical equipment and reducing the need for frequent replacements and associated manufacturing emissions.

Research and Development: AI can analyze vast datasets to identify and develop sustainable healthcare solutions, from bio-based medical materials to eco-friendly sterilization processes.

Policy and Regulation: AI can inform policy decisions and regulations around sustainable healthcare practices, promoting green standards and accountability across the healthcare system.

4. Embracing a Holistic Approach:

Lifecycle Assessment: It's crucial to consider the entire lifecycle of AI in healthcare, from data collection and algorithm development to deployment and maintenance, ensuring all stages are optimized for sustainability.

Collaboration and Transparency: Collaboration among clinicians, engineers, ecologists, and policymakers is key to developing and implementing effective green AI solutions. Transparency and responsible development practices foster trust and public acceptance.

Continuous Improvement: As AI technology evolves, it's vital to continually assess and improve its environmental impact, adopting new strategies and adapting existing ones to ensure ongoing progress towards sustainability.

By actively pursuing these strategies and prioritizing environmental responsibility, AI can transform from a potential environmental burden to a powerful force for good in healthcare. Remember, making AI a net positive contributor to environmental sustainability isn't just a technological challenge; it's a social, ethical, and economic imperative. By leveraging the power of AI with a green mindset, we can pave the way for a healthier planet and a more sustainable future for healthcare for generations to come. Let's not merely treat symptoms; let's address the root cause of the environmental impact of AI in healthcare. Let's turn AI into a catalyst for change, one green innovation at a time.

Chapter 13

Measuring Impact and Success

Artificial intelligence (AI) has cast its spell on the world, promising a future where machines outthink humans, revolutionize industries, and cure diseases. But amidst the fanfare, an essential question lingers in the shadows: how do we know if AI is truly achieving its promises, or are we merely lost in a labyrinth of algorithms? The answer lies in a crucial yet often overlooked aspect – measuring the impact and success of AI.

Traditionally, success in AI has been measured through the technical lens of accuracy rates, data processing speed, and impressive demonstrations of superhuman ability. While these feats are undoubtedly remarkable, they offer a distorted picture, akin to judging a book by its cover. To truly understand the impact of AI, we must venture beyond the technical marvel and into the human-centric heart of the matter.

Imagine a self-driving car boasting near-perfect accident avoidance in controlled environments. Its algorithm accuracy is impeccable, its processing speed unmatched. Yet, if its real-world deployment leads to increased traffic congestion, exacerbates social inequalities by limiting mobility, or raises privacy concerns, then can we truly call it a success? Clearly, the mere absence of crashes is not enough. We must consider the broader impact of AI on human well-being, social equity, and ethical implications.

In the realm of medicine and healthcare, the need for measuring AI's impact becomes even more critical. Lives hang in the balance, and decisions made by AI algorithms can have profound consequences for patients. Therefore, simply relying on technical metrics like diagnostic accuracy or prediction is akin to treating a symptom without addressing the root cause.

Consider these scenarios:

- An AI-powered diagnostic tool boasts near-perfect accuracy in detecting cancer, but it exacerbates existing healthcare disparities by disproportionately misdiagnosing people of color. This demonstrates the need for not just high accuracy, but also equitable outcomes and ethical considerations.
- A treatment algorithm optimizes medication dosages for maximum efficacy, but it leads to increased side effects and patient discomfort. This highlights the importance of measuring not just clinical outcomes, but also patient well-being and quality of life.
- A surgical robot performs flawlessly in operating rooms, but its implementation disrupts established workflows, alienates surgeons, and hinders communication between humans and machines. This underscores the need for seamless integration of AI into existing healthcare practices, prioritizing collaboration over automation.

Therefore, to assess AI's impact, we must shift our lens from technology to humanity. Here are some crucial considerations:

- Shifting Focus: From Metrics to Meaning: Move beyond cold statistics like performance benchmarks and embrace metrics that reflect human well-being, individual empowerment, and social equity. Measuring changes in healthcare outcomes, environmental impact, and access to opportunities paints a more accurate picture of success than sheer algorithmic prowess.

- Long-Term Vision: Avoid the allure of short-term gains like increased profits or productivity. Consider the potential long-term consequences, both positive and negative, of AI implementation. Is it contributing to a sustainable future, or merely exacerbating existing inequalities? Responsible AI demands a holistic vision that prioritizes lasting benefits over fleeting gains.
- Transparency and Accountability: AI algorithms and data practices must be demystified, open to scrutiny, and understandable to the public. Without transparency, trust in AI crumbles, hindering its potential to truly benefit society.
- Collaboration and Diverse Perspectives: Evaluating AI should not be a solitary intellectual exercise conducted in ivory towers. Diverse stakeholders – researchers, ethicists, policymakers, and affected communities – must collaborate to ensure AI is developed and deployed with a profound understanding of its impact on all.
- Human well-being and quality of life: Does AI improve lives by alleviating suffering, empowering individuals, or fostering greater equity?
- Social and ethical implications: Does AI exacerbate existing biases, violate privacy rights, or contribute to job displacement?
- Sustainability and ecological impact: Does AI promote responsible resource management, mitigate environmental harm, or contribute to a more sustainable future?

Measuring the impact and success of AI is not just a technical exercise; it's a vital step towards ensuring that this powerful technology is used responsibly and ethically for the benefit of all. By taking the time to measure and understand the impact of AI, we can pave the way for a future where AI fosters progress, well-being, and a more equitable world. Measuring the impact and success of AI is crucial for several reasons:

1. Ensuring responsible development and deployment: Without proper evaluation, we risk unintended consequences like biases, discrimination, and privacy violations. Measuring impact helps us

identify ethical problems and course-correct to ensure AI benefits everyone.
2. Optimizing performance and ROI: Evaluating AI's effectiveness helps us understand which applications are producing valuable results and where improvements are needed. This allows us to prioritize resources, refine algorithms, and maximize return on investment.
3. Building trust and public acceptance: Without evidence of positive impact, it's difficult to convince people that AI is safe and beneficial. Measuring success helps demonstrate the tangible benefits of AI to build public trust and encourage wider adoption.
4. Guiding future development: Evaluating past successes and failures informs future research and development efforts. By understanding what works and what doesn't, we can focus on developing responsible and beneficial AI applications that truly address real-world needs.
5. Holding developers and stakeholders accountable: Measuring impact ensures transparency and accountability throughout the AI development and deployment process. This helps foster responsible practices and discourages the use of AI for unethical purposes.
6. Contributing to a broader understanding of AI: By systematically evaluating AI's impact across various applications and fields, we can gain valuable insights into its potential and limitations. This knowledge can inform discussions on AI ethics, policy, and governance.

Developing a robust framework for measuring AI's impact in healthcare requires a multifaceted approach. Here are some key considerations:

1. Clinical outcomes: Measuring disease detection rates, treatment efficacy, and improved patient survival provides tangible evidence of success.
2. Patient experience: Surveys, interviews, and focus groups can shed light on patient understanding, trust, and engagement with AI-powered care.

3. Workflow efficiency: Time saved, reduced workloads, and improved data access can demonstrate the practical benefits of AI integration.
4. Ethical considerations: Regular audits for bias, adherence to data privacy regulations, and transparency measures must be established.
5. Economic impact: Cost savings, resource allocation optimization, and potential economic benefits for both healthcare providers and patients should be evaluated.
6. Enhancing Healthcare Provider Productivity: A key metric for AI success in healthcare is its effect on provider productivity. AI can streamline labor-intensive tasks, freeing healthcare professionals to concentrate on patient care. Metrics like increased patient throughput or reduced administrative burdens are indicators of AI's effectiveness. For instance:

   - AI-driven diagnostic tools aid in faster, more accurate patient assessments, leading to improved treatment plans.
   - AI applications in administrative tasks, like patient scheduling or records management, can significantly reduce the time spent on paperwork.

7. Accelerating Clinical Decision-Making: AI's ability to swiftly analyze complex medical data can expedite clinical decision-making. Success in this area can be measured by the reduced duration from diagnosis to treatment initiation. For example:

   - AI systems that analyze medical imaging or lab results can provide quicker insights, leading to faster patient management decisions.
   - Real-time data analysis tools can alert healthcare providers to emerging patient issues, allowing for prompt intervention.

8. Tracking AI Utilization and Adoption: Monitoring how healthcare professionals use and adopt AI systems offers insights into their effectiveness. Metrics like user count, application frequency, and

direct feedback highlight AI's acceptance and utility in healthcare settings. Further, assessing AI's impact on key performance indicators (KPIs) such as patient outcomes, cost efficiency, or treatment efficacy is essential.

- ➢ Usage analytics can reveal the extent of AI integration in various hospital departments or clinics.
- ➢ Patient care coordination tools powered by AI can be evaluated based on usage rates and feedback from healthcare teams.

9. Assessing Accuracy and Clinical Performance: The precision and reliability of AI algorithms are crucial in healthcare. Evaluating these using metrics like accuracy, sensitivity, and specificity, especially in diagnostic AI tools, is vital for ensuring patient safety and effective treatments.

- ➢ AI systems used in pathology or radiology can be assessed for their accuracy in detecting abnormalities compared to traditional methods.
- ➢ The performance of AI in predictive analytics, like forecasting patient deterioration, can be measured against established clinical benchmarks.

10. Return on Investment (ROI) Analysis: Evaluating the financial implications of AI in healthcare is critical. ROI analysis involves weighing the costs of AI implementation and maintenance against benefits such as operational efficiencies, reduced readmission rates, and improved patient care quality.

11. Gathering User Feedback and Patient Satisfaction: Collecting feedback from healthcare providers and patients is essential in measuring AI's success. Surveys and direct feedback methods can gauge perceptions about AI's utility, ease of use, and overall impact on patient care. High levels of satisfaction and positive feedback are indicative of successful AI integration.

Measuring the success of AI in healthcare encompasses a range of factors, from provider productivity and decision-making efficiency to clinical accuracy and financial viability. Defining clear metrics and objectives from the outset is crucial for effective evaluation. By systematically measuring AI's impact, healthcare organizations can optimize AI initiatives, leading to enhanced patient care and operational excellence. Remember, the true success of AI lies not in chasing the highest accuracy rate or generating the most viral video, but in its ability to improve lives, empower individuals, and contribute to a more equitable and sustainable world. Let us move beyond the technical metrics and embrace the human-centric lens of impact, for it is in understanding the true consequences of AI that we unlock its transformative potential.

Conclusion

As we close the pages of "Code to Care," we find ourselves at a crossroads. On one path lies the alluring but precarious promise of AI: personalized medicine, streamlined workflows, and revolutionary cures. On the other lies the responsibility to navigate this path with prudence, ensuring that technology heals, not harms. This book has been your compass, guiding you, the healthcare leader, through the intricacies of implementing responsible AI, transforming "code" into compassionate care.

You've traversed the promise and peril of AI in healthcare, laying a foundation of responsible development built on fairness, transparency, and accountability. You've learned to orchestrate a 360-degree approach, aligning your organization and governance models with AI's needs. You've grappled with risk assessment and mitigation, securing your digital frontier against threats that could eclipse progress.

But responsible AI is not just about defense; it's about exploration. We've ventured into the realm of generative AI, where possibilities bloom like digital roses, offering personalized treatment plans and groundbreaking drug discovery. And lest we forget the human touch, we've learned from the airline industry, where humans and AI collaborate in a harmonious symphony, guiding patients to recovery just as pilots navigate turbulent skies.

Finally, we've embraced the mantle of Green AI, ensuring that our technological advances do not come at the cost of our planet's health.

Remember, a sustainable future for healthcare can only thrive when code and care intertwine, blossoming into a world where technology heals not just bodies, but the environment that sustains them.

As you step away from this book, let its lessons resonate within you. Be the champion of responsible AI, the leader who fosters trust and ensures technology serves humanity. Build a healthcare system where algorithms hum in harmony with compassion, where data sparks insights that illuminate personalized treatment paths, and where every line of code whispers a promise of care.

Remember, the future of healthcare isn't written in algorithms alone; it's written in the choices we make today. Choose responsibility, choose collaboration, choose humanity. Let "Code to Care" be not just a guide, but a springboard, propelling you forward towards a future where AI enhances healthcare, not replaces it, where technology becomes a powerful ally in the age-old human endeavor of healing.

For it is in this act of responsible implementation, in this harmonious blend of code and care, that we finally fulfill the true promise of AI in healthcare: not just to revolutionize treatment, but to revolutionize ourselves, becoming the architects of a future where technology blossoms into care, and healthcare thrives for generations to come.

As leaders in healthcare, the journey towards responsible AI implementation is ongoing. It requires continuous learning, adaptation, and vigilance. This book has aimed to equip you with the knowledge, strategies, and insights to navigate this complex landscape effectively. The future of healthcare, shaped by AI, holds unparalleled opportunities for improvement in patient care and operational efficiency. However, it is up to us, the leaders, to ensure that this technology is harnessed with responsibility, ethical integrity, and a relentless focus on the human element at the heart of healthcare.

In embracing responsible AI, we are not just adopting a new set of tools; we are pioneering a new era in healthcare – one that holds the promise of enhanced patient outcomes, operational excellence, and a deeper understanding of the complex tapestry of human health. Let us step forward with confidence, guided by the principles and lessons of "Code to Care."

About the Author

Rubin Pillay, MD, PhD is a dynamic and visionary leader at the forefront of transforming healthcare through innovative strategies and digital health technologies. With a wealth of expertise in healthcare management, technology, and entrepreneurship, Dr. Pillay has become a trusted voice in the industry, inspiring change and driving impactful solutions. As an accomplished author, speaker, and academic, Dr. Pillay combines his extensive knowledge with a deep understanding of the challenges faced by the healthcare sector. His unique perspective and forward-thinking approach have made him a sought-after advisor for healthcare organizations, policymakers, and industry leaders around the globe. Dr. Pillay's passion lies in harnessing the potential of digital health to create sustainable, patient-centered healthcare systems. With a keen focus on achieving the seven transformative "zeros" in healthcare, he brings to light the power of digital technology to drive positive change. His thought-provoking insights challenge conventional practices, ignite innovation, and inspire healthcare professionals to envision a brighter future. Beyond his academic and professional achievements, Dr. Pillay is known for his unwavering commitment to improving patient outcomes, fostering collaboration, and tackling healthcare disparities. He is driven by a deep sense of purpose, aiming to create a healthcare landscape that is accessible, efficient, and sustainable for all. Dr. Pillay's influence extends far beyond the written word. He is an engaging and captivating speaker, delivering impactful keynote addresses and presentations that leave audiences inspired and motivated. With a natural ability to connect with diverse audiences, he empowers others to embrace change, seize opportunities, and drive meaningful transformation in their own healthcare organizations.

As the healthcare landscape continues to evolve rapidly, Dr. Rubin Pillay remains at the forefront of innovation, leading the charge towards a future where technology, compassion, and sustainability converge. His unwavering dedication, expertise, and visionary mindset make him a true catalyst for positive change in healthcare. Whether you're a healthcare professional, policymaker, or an individual passionate about improving healthcare, Rubin Pillay is a name that should be on your radar. Prepare to be inspired, challenged, and enlightened by his unique perspectives as he paves the way towards a brighter and more sustainable future for us all.

www.ingramcontent.com/pod-product-compliance
Lightning Source LLC
Chambersburg PA
CBHW020638220526
45464CB00001B/194